# AUDITORY COMPREHENSION
*Clinical and Experimental Studies
with the Token Test*

PERSPECTIVES IN
NEUROLINGUISTICS AND PSYCHOLINGUISTICS

Harry A. Whitaker, Series Editor
DEPARTMENT OF PSYCHOLOGY
THE UNIVERSITY OF ROCHESTER
ROCHESTER, NEW YORK

HAIGANOOSH WHITAKER and HARRY A. WHITAKER (Eds.).
Studies in Neurolinguistics, Volumes 1, 2, and 3

NORMAN J. LASS (Ed.). Contemporary Issues in Experimental Phonetics

JASON W. BROWN. Mind, Brain, and Consciousness: The Neuropsychology of Cognition

SIDNEY J. SEGALOWITZ and FREDERIC A. GRUBER (Eds.). Language Development and Neurological Theory

SUSAN CURTISS. Genie: A Psycholinguistic Study of a Modern-Day "Wild Child"

JOHN MACNAMARA (Ed.). Language Learning and Thought

I. M. SCHLESINGER and LILA NAMIR (Eds.). Sign Language of the Deaf: Psychological, Linguistic, and Sociological Perspectives

WILLIAM C. RITCHIE (Ed.). Second Language Acquisition Research: Issues and Implications

PATRICIA SIPLE (Ed.). Understanding Language through Sign Language Research

MARTIN L. ALBERT and LORAINE K. OBLER. The Bilingual Brain: Neurophysiological and Neurolinguistic Aspects of Bilingualism

HAIGANOOSH WHITAKER and HARRY A. WHITAKER (Eds.). Studies in Neurolinguistics, Volume 4

TALMY GIVON. On Understanding Grammar

CHARLES J. FILLMORE, DANIEL KEMPLER and WILLIAM S-Y. WANG (Eds.). Individual Differences in Language Ability and Language Behavior

JEANNINE HERRON (Ed.). Neuropsychology of Left-Handedness

FRANCOIS BOLLER and MAUREEN DENNIS (Eds.). Auditory Comprehension: Clinical and Experimental Studies with the Token Test

*In preparation*

R. W. RIEBER (Ed.). Language Development and Aphasia in Children: New Essays and a Translation of "Kindersprache und Aphasie" by Emil Fröschels

# AUDITORY COMPREHENSION

*Clinical and Experimental Studies with the Token Test*

Edited by

## FRANÇOIS BOLLER

*Neurobehavior Research and Clinical Center*
*University of Pittsburgh School of Medicine*
*Pittsburgh, Pennsylvania*

## MAUREEN DENNIS

*Department of Psychology*
*The Hospital for Sick Children*
*Toronto, Ontario, Canada*

1979

ACADEMIC PRESS
*A Subsidiary of Harcourt Brace Jovanovich, Publishers*
New York   London   Toronto   Sydney   San Francisco

COPYRIGHT © 1979, BY ACADEMIC PRESS, INC.
ALL RIGHTS RESERVED.
NO PART OF THIS PUBLICATION MAY BE REPRODUCED OR
TRANSMITTED IN ANY FORM OR BY ANY MEANS, ELECTRONIC
OR MECHANICAL, INCLUDING PHOTOCOPY, RECORDING, OR ANY
INFORMATION STORAGE AND RETRIEVAL SYSTEM, WITHOUT
PERMISSION IN WRITING FROM THE PUBLISHER.

ACADEMIC PRESS, INC.
111 Fifth Avenue, New York, New York 10003

*United Kingdom Edition published by*
ACADEMIC PRESS, INC. (LONDON) LTD.
24/28 Oval Road, London NW1 7DX

Library of Congress Cataloging in Publication Data
Main entry under title:

Auditory comprehension.

(Perspectives in neurolinguistics and psycholin-
guistics)
Bibliography: p.
1. Token Test.  I. Boller, Francois. II. Dennis,
Maureen.
RC425.A92              616.8'552'075        79-22510
ISBN 0-12-111650-6

PRINTED IN THE UNITED STATES OF AMERICA

79 80 81 82     9 8 7 6 5 4 3 2 1

# Contents

List of Contributors ix
Preface xi

## I  THE TOKEN TEST AND ITS PRECURSORS

1  Introduction: Testing for Comprehension: A Short History of Comprehension Tests up to the Token Test  3
FRANÇOIS BOLLER

2  The Token Test: A Sensitive Test to Detect Receptive Disturbances in Aphasics  15
ENNIO De RENZI AND LUIGI A. VIGNOLO

## II  REVISED TESTS

3   A Shortened Version of the Token Test                                33
    ENNIO De RENZI

4   Components of Auditory Comprehension:
    Analysis of Errors in a Revised Token Test                           45
    JAMES L. MACK AND FRANÇOIS BOLLER

5   Turning Tokens into Things:
    Linguistic and Mnestic Aspects
    of the Initial Sections of the Token Test                            71
    RUTH LESSER

## III  NEUROLINGUISTIC ANALYSIS

6   Lexical, Syntactic, and Semantic Aspects of
    the Token Test: A Linguistic Taxonomy                                89
    HARRY A. WHITAKER AND HAIGANOOSH WHITAKER

7   Performance of Aphasic Patients in Visual
    versus Auditory Presentation of the Token Test:
    Demonstration of a Supramodal Deficit                               107
    KLAUS POECK AND WOLFGANG HARTJE

## IV  CLINICAL APPLICATIONS

8   Nondiagnostic Uses of the Token Test                                117
    AUDREY L. HOLLAND AND JANET L. WHITNEY

9   Use of the Token Test with Children:
    Two Contrasting Socioeconomic Groups                                125
    J. DOUGLAS NOLL AND NORMAN J. LASS

## V CEREBRAL LOCALIZATION OF TOKEN TEST PERFORMANCE

**10** Long-Term Stability of Hemispheric Scores on the Token Test Following Brain Bisection and Hemidecortication    135
ERAN ZAIDEL

**11** Lesions Underlying Defective Performances on the Token Test: A CT Scan Study    161
LUIGI A. VIGNOLO

## VI RESEARCH DIRECTIONS

**12** Epilogue: Research Applications and Directions    171
MAUREEN DENNIS

References    181

SUBJECT INDEX    189

## List of Contributors

*Numbers in parentheses indicate the pages on which the authors' contributions begin.*

FRANÇOIS BOLLER (3, 45), Neurobehavior Research and Clinical Center, University of Pittsburgh School of Medicine, Pittsburgh, Pennsylvania 15261

MAUREEN DENNIS (171), Department of Psychology, The Hospital for Sick Children, Toronto, Ontario, M5G 1X8 Canada

ENNIO DE RENZI (15, 33), Department of Neurology, University of Modena, Via del Pozzo, 7I, Modena 41100, Italy

WOLFGANG HARTJE (107), Abteilung Neurologie, Rheinisch-Westfälische Technische Hochschule Aachen, 5100 Aachen, Goethestrasse 27-29 West Germany

AUDREY L. HOLLAND (117), Department of Speech, University of Pittsburgh, Pittsburgh, Pennsylvania 15260

NORMAN J. LASS (125), Department of Speech Pathology and Audiology, West Virginia University, Morgantown, West Virginia 26505

RUTH LESSER (71), School of Education, University of Newcastle upon Tyne, Newcastle upon Tyne NE1 7RU, England

JAMES L. MACK (45), Division of Neurology, Case Western Reserve University School of Medicine, Cleveland, Ohio 44106

J. DOUGLAS NOLL (125), Department of Audiology and Speech Sciences, Purdue University, Lafayette, Indiana 47907

KLAUS POECK (107), Abteilung Neurologie, Rheinisch-Westfälische Technische Hochschule Aachen, 5100 Aachen, Goethestrasse 27-29, West Germany

LUIGI A. VIGNOLO (15, 161), Clinica Neurologica, Università di Milano, Milano, Italy

HAIGANOOSH WHITAKER (89), Department of Psychology, University of Rochester, Rochester, New York 14627

HARRY A. WHITAKER (89), Department of Psychology, University of Rochester, Rochester, New York 14627

JANET L. WHITNEY (117), Department of Speech, University of Pittsburgh, Pittsburgh, Pennsylvania 15260

ERAN ZAIDEL (135), Division of Biology, California Institute of Technology, Pasadena, California 92215

# Preface

The Token Test consists of commands of progressive complexity in which a subject is requested to touch or move tokens of different shape, color, and, sometimes, size. The ease of its application, its readily quantifiable results, and its sensitivity even to subtle forms of aphasia have made it a very popular tool for the clinical diagnosis of the comprehension impairment that is frequently part of language disorders. The Token Test has also contributed significantly to the considerable surge of research in auditory comprehension witnessed in recent years. Almost two decades after its introduction, we felt that there was need for a book that brings together recent contributions from the two original authors of the Token Test, as well as contributions by several others who have used the test extensively. The book emphasizes both the clinical and the research aspects of the test, with particular stress on its clinical indications and on the insight it has provided to comprehension disorders, aphasia, language, and to brain and behavior relationships.

This volume is intended for all those who are exposed to patients with language disorders, particularly clinicians who diagnose or treat aphasics and for researchers in the field of human neuropsychology. It will therefore be of interest to persons of widely diverse backgrounds, including neurologists, psychiatrists, speech pathologists, and other clinicians as well as neurolinguists and neuropsychologists.

Included in this work is a review of the historical background of the Token Test, a reprint of DeRenzi and Vignolo's original 1962 article, and several current variations and applications introduced for either clinical or research purpose. These include shorter versions of the Token Test, modifications of the stimuli used as the mode of presentation, and an analysis of performance by each cerebral hemisphere. The book also deals with the linguistic implications of the Token Test and with the relations between test impairment and anatomical lesions. It concludes with a critical view of the present status of the test and with suggestions for future research. The chapters are grouped into six sections: the test and its precursors, revised tests, neurolinguistic analysis, clinical applications, cerebral localization of Token Test performance, and research directions.

This work is the written counterpart, but not the proceedings, of a symposium that was held at the Annual Meeting of the American Speech and Hearing Association in Chicago in 1977, and we express our thanks to the Program Committee of ASHA for the help they provided in organizing it. We are indebted to Oxford University Press for their permission to reprint DeRenzi and Vignolo's original article from *Brain*. Figures 1.2, 1.3, and 1.5 were reprinted through the courtesy of Charles C Thomas and Arnold Publishing Co. Finally, we wish to thank the staff of Academic Press for their invaluable help in the production of this volume.

# I
## THE TOKEN TEST AND ITS PRECURSORS

# 1

## Introduction: Testing for Comprehension: A Short History of Comprehension Tests up to the Token Test

FRANÇOIS BOLLER

DeRenzi and Vignolo published their original description of the Token Test in 1962. In the intervening years, the Token Test has become an essential tool in the assessment of aphasia and has been the subject of many experimental papers. The present book reviews the state of the art of both clinical and experimental applications of the test. By way of introduction, it may be of interest to review briefly the early tests which led to the development of the Token Test. We will not describe them in detail, since many are of little use today and because information about them appears in the original literature and in other recent reviews (Benton, 1973; Boller, Kim, & Mack, 1977; Boller, 1978). Instead we will attempt to follow the lines of thought of different authors and extract from them the ideas which have led to the construction of the Token Test.

Early descriptions of aphasia were based on observations and case reports by investigators with alert minds but little proclivity toward objective, systematized testing. It was only in later years that aphasiologists began to use special batteries of tests which sometimes included comprehension tests. The Frenchman Achille-Adrien Proust (1834–1903), uncle of the famous writer, is sometimes credited with developing the earliest special test for comprehension testing (1872). In this test, the patient was asked to raise his fingers as many times as there were syllables in the name of an object shown by the examiner. However, it is questionable whether such a test (assuming that a patient is able to understand what he must do) can really be considered an index of comprehension.

Two early contributions to comprehension testing are found in the German literature. Grashey (1885) published a picture test designed to evaluate object recognition. Soon afterwards, Rieger (1888–1890) was

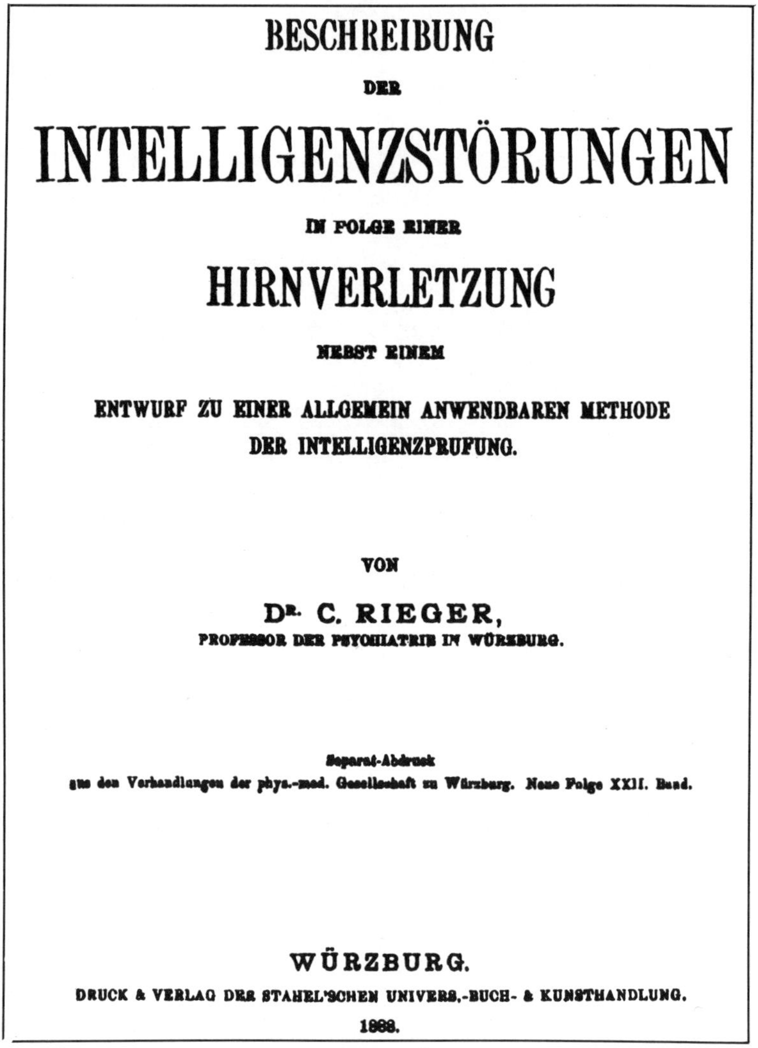

**BESCHREIBUNG**

DER

# INTELLIGENZSTÖRUNGEN

IN FOLGE EINER

## HIRNVERLETZUNG

NEBST EINEM

ENTWURF ZU EINER ALLGEMEIN ANWENDBAREN METHODE
DER INTELLIGENZPRÜFUNG.

VON

**DR. C. RIEGER,**
PROFESSOR DER PSYCHIATRIE IN WÜRZBURG.

Separat-Abdruck
aus den Verhandlungen der phys.-med. Gesellschaft zu Würzburg. Neue Folge XXII. Band.

**WÜRZBURG.**
DRUCK & VERLAG DER STAHEL'SCHEN UNIVERS.-BUCH- & KUNSTHANDLUNG.
1888.

**FIGURE 1.1.** *Title page of Rieger's Book (1888). (Courtesy Arthur L. Benton.)*

probably the first to publish a large-scale battery which could test both intellectual and language functions in brain-damaged patients (see Figure 1.1).

After Rieger, several aphasiologists began to use the method which is now the standard for assessing comprehension and, in fact, neuropsychological deficits of any kind: Deficiency levels were determined by testing subjects with items of increasing complexity.

Comprehension-test batteries were proposed by Pierre Marie (see Figure 1.2) (1906), Liepmann (1908), and Goldstein (1948), among others. One of the tests of Marie's battery, which he considered the most difficult, deserves particular mention here because it is one of the few

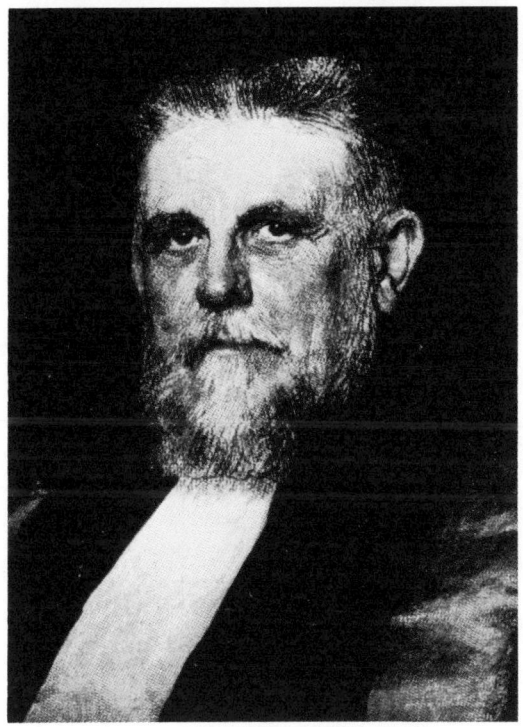

**FIGURE 1.2.** *Portrait and autograph of Pierre Marie. (Reprinted from W. Haymaker (Ed.), The Founders of Neurology, Springfield, Ill.: Charles C Thomas, Publisher, 1972, with permission.)*

comprehension tests of those early years to have achieved and retained notoriety. Marie's Paper Test consists simply of giving a patient a complex sequential command: "Here on this table are three pieces of paper of different sizes; give me the largest one, crumple the middle-sized one and throw it on the floor; as for the smaller one, put it in your pocket."

The merit of this test is its extreme ease of application. It can be administered at the patient's bedside, requires no special material, and is easy to quantify. It was included as part of the battery of Goldstein (1948) and Weisenburg and McBride (1935), but these authors did not describe its use with either aphasics or normals. Is Marie's Paper Test actually a reliable measure of auditory comprehension in aphasia?

Boller and Vignolo (1966) used the Paper Test with four groups of subjects: normal controls, right brain-damaged (RBD) patients, left brain-damaged (LBD) patients without evidence of aphasia, and LBD patients with mild receptive deficits. A score of one was given for correct performance on each of the three steps. Table 1.1 shows the scores obtained by the four groups. As can be seen, the test is very easy for normals (only one failed) and for the RBD and the nonaphasic subjects (only two failed in each group). Of the LBD aphasic group, 29 out of 34 (85%) also showed no impairment. Without repetition of commands, only 65% of the aphasic subjects performed without error, but the performance of the other three groups also suffered. There was no significant difference between normal and aphasic performance either with or without repeated commands, and the test discriminated poorly between groups.

**TABLE 1.1**
*Scores of Four Experimental Groups on Marie's Paper Test*[a]

| Scores | Controls | | Brain-damaged patients | | | | | |
|---|---|---|---|---|---|---|---|---|
| | | | Right | | Left | | | |
| | | | | | Nonaphasic | | Aphasic | |
| | (N=31) | | (N=30) | | (N=26) | | (N=34) | |
| | E | S | E | S | E | S | E | S |
| 3 | 15 | 15 | 18 | 10 | 13 | 11 | 13 | 15 |
| 2 | | | 1 | | 1 | 1 | 2 | 1 |
| 1 | 1 | | 1 | | | | 2 | |
| 0 | | | | | | | 1 | |

[a] E = patients with elementary education (less than 6 years); S = patients with secondary or superior education (more than 6 years); dotted line (···) represents normal cut-off score.

# INTRODUCTION: TESTING FOR COMPREHENSION

It may be worth emphasizing, however, that the aphasic group was selected by Boller and Vignolo (1966) for the presence of only minimal or mild comprehension disturbance. Results from giving the Paper Test to an unselected sample of aphasics are not available.

In his book, *Aphasia and Kindred Disorders of Speech,* Head (1926) (see Figure 1.3) described a series of tests used in his examination of aphasics. They included naming and recognition of objects (pointing to an object on command); naming and recognition of colors; The Man–Cat–Dog Test (an easy reading and writing test); and the Clock Test, involving setting the hands of the clock and telling the time. More relevant to auditory comprehension are the Coin in Bowl Test, and the Hand–

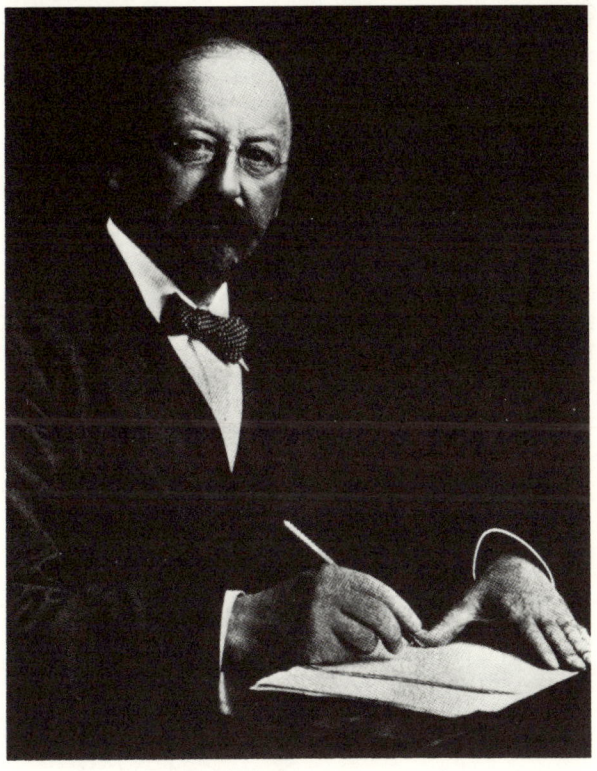

**FIGURE 1.3.** *Portrait and autograph of Henry Head. (Reprinted from W. Haymaker (Ed.),* The Founders of Neurology, *Springfield, Ill.: Charles C Thomas, Publisher, 1972, with permission.)*

Eye-Ear Test. In the former test, four bowls or saucers are set upon a table and a penny is placed in front of each. The patient is then asked to place the pennies in the bowls during a series of commands. In the latter test, the patient is requested to touch an eye or an ear with one or the other hand (Figure 1.4).

The tests proposed by Head (1926) for testing oral comprehension, particularly the Hand-Eye-Ear test, have been used by several examiners (Pearson, Alpers, & Weisenburg, 1928; Quadfasel, 1931; Goldstein, 1948; Orgass & Poeck, 1969). Most authors suggest that failure to perform the task in the Hand-Eye-Ear Test correctly may be due not only to aphasia but also to impairments of visuo-spatial ability and to limited intelligence. However, even normal adults of superior intelligence may fail on this and other tests in Head's battery (Pearson *et al.*, 1928). On the other hand, Orgass and Poeck (1969), using a series of verbal tests in an effort to identify those with the most specific diagnostic value for

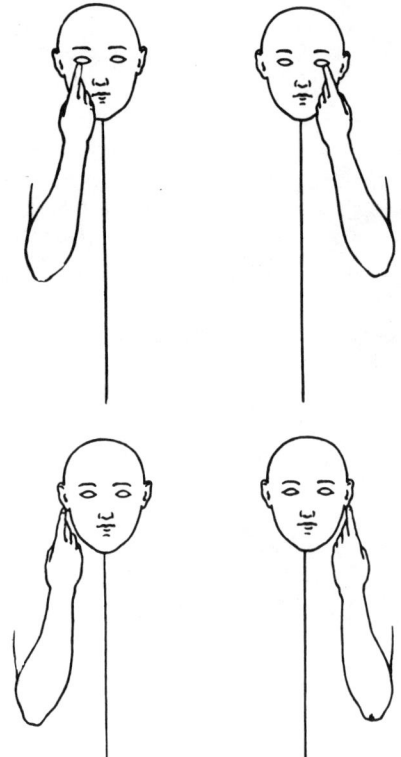

**FIGURE 1.4.** *Sample from Head's Hand-Eye-Ear Test. (From Head, 1926.)*

aphasia, found that the four tests best able to discriminate between aphasic and nonaphasic brain-damaged subjects included the Hand–Eye–Ear Test. (The other three tests were a Verbal IQ, an Arithmetic Calculation Test, and the Token Test.) It must be noted, however, that Orgass and Poeck (1969) used their own version of Head's test. Therefore, it is possible that the discrepancy between their findings and those of other writers is due to methodological differences. Overall, it seems difficult to determine what aspects of Head's test account for the aphasic's impaired response to it and therefore also difficult to judge the extent to which the test may be considered a measure of comprehension.

A series of tests described by Weisenburg and McBride (1935) may be considered the first of the modern aphasia batteries. In an introduction, "Psychological examination for aphasic patients, a discussion of the essential requirements," they outline some of the principles used in the construction of this battery. They point out that a battery for aphasia should cover all the performances which may be disturbed. As many as possible of the tests selected for a preliminary examination should be standardized, so that the results obtained by one investigator can be compared with those obtained by another. At the same time, the standard tests must be capable of being altered to throw more light on unusual difficulties. Thus, although Weisenburg and McBride realized the importance of standardization, they emphasized that the fundamental purpose of a language test is to provide a thorough analysis of the individual patient's language behavior, including his method of work, the factors which appear to cause his failures, and the nature of the responses he finally achieves. They felt that the least complicated tests were most likely to provide such specific information. Weisenburg and McBride also pointed out the need for adequate testing of comprehension of oral and written material in a comparable manner. Finally, because of the great variability in the performance of aphasics, they emphasized that tasks must be of a sufficient range of difficulty in order to be applied to all patients.

The tests Weisenburg and McBride chose to assess comprehension emphasize general intelligence and are often difficult even for normal subjects. The authors intended to use tests that would achieve a broad dispersion of scores so as to permit the comparison of patients with comprehension deficits of widely varying severity. As a result, these tests are often difficult to interpret in terms of a patient's specific linguistic abilities.

Ombredane (see Figure 1.5) made an important contribution to comprehension testing when he described (1951) an assessment technique that stressed the role of particular types of words in identifying

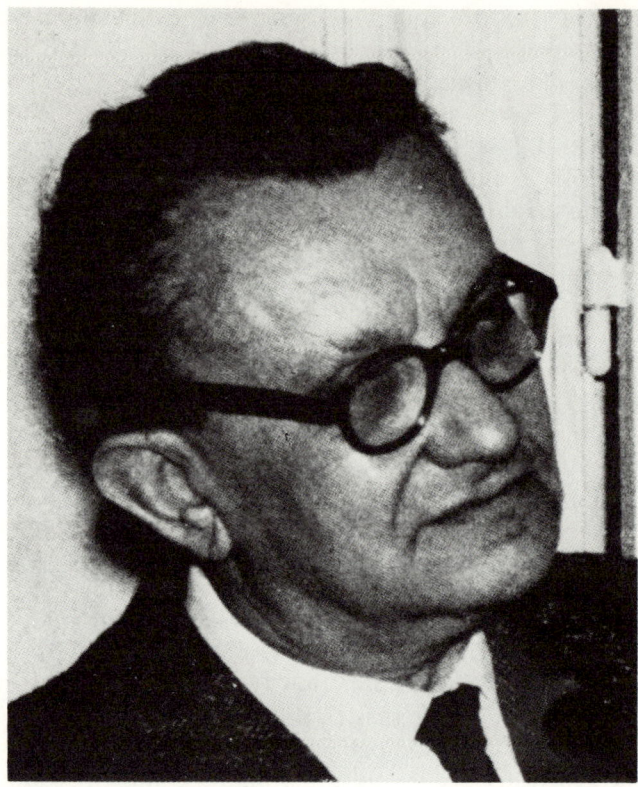

**FIGURE 1.5.** *André Ombredane. (Reprinted from M. Critchley,* Aphasiology, *London: Arnold, 1970, with permission.)*

comprehension problems. In the Cat and Chair Test (see Figure 1.6) six cards are displayed in front of the patient, each showing a cat either on, before, to the right of, below, behind, or to the left of a chair. The patient is asked to point to the card corresponding to a sentence spoken by the examiner that describes, by the use of a certain preposition, the positional relationship of the cat to the chair. In the Pencils Test, the patient is presented with two groups of pencils, one to his left and one to his right. Each group contains a long red pencil, a short red pencil, a long blue pencil, and a short blue pencil. The patient is then instructed to select from the eight pencils the one described aloud by the examiner, for example, "the long red pencil on your right." Thus, his ability to comprehend and utilize descriptive attributes and positional relationships is evaluated in a contest seemingly unrelated to high general intellectual ability, although, of course, attentional deficits could well influence the patient's performance. These two tests are somewhat reminiscent of Head's Coin in Bowl Test and seem clearly to be precursors of DeRenzi and Vignolo's Token Test.

In the construction of the Token Test, the contribution of psycholinguistics, although it centered on normal language rather than on aphasia, was also taken into account. Psycholinguists (see, for example, Miller, 1951) have pointed out that in any natural language more symbols are used to encode a message than are theoretically necessary. In other words, ordinary language is highly redundant. The main advantage of redundancy is, of course, to reduce errors. However, it is theoretically possible to construct messages so low in redundancy that the comprehension of each component unit of the message is necessary for understanding. It would thus appear that the lower the redundancy, a more precise assessment of comprehension would be possible with less difficulty.

The following chapters include a reprint of DeRenzi and Vignolo's original 1962 article and deal with several different aspects of the Token Test. According to most authors who have used it, the Token Test does not lose its diagnostic power when shorter versions are used. After reviewing some of the criteria used in the construction of the original

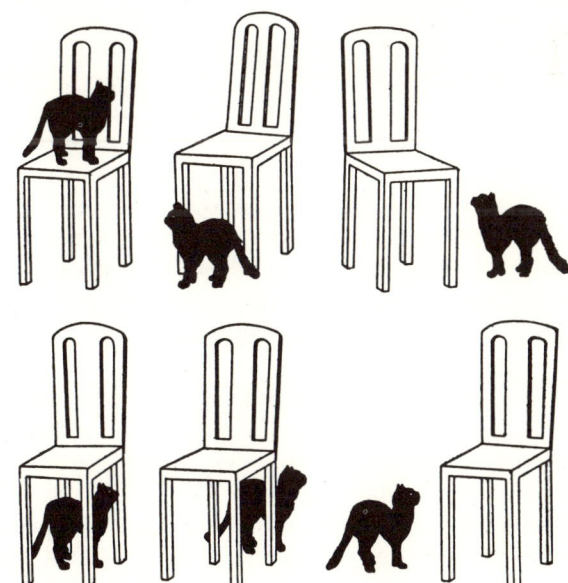

**FIGURE 1.6.** *Ombredane's Cat and Chair Test. (From Ombredane, 1951.)*

Token Test, De Renzi presents his results on a 36-item version of the test, shorter than the original 61-item version. The "hit rate" of this new version is 5% false positive, 7% false negative, a rate that roughly corresponds to that of the longer version.

One of the purposes of this book is to show that, in addition to its clinical purpose, the Token Test can be used to clarify neurolinguistic issues concerning comprehension. One approach is to use modified commands which is exemplified in the next two chapters. Mack and Boller present their analysis of errors made by aphasic and nonaphasic patients, both in the "classical" Token Test and in a revised version of the test. Their data support a qualitative difference between the comprehension deficits of nonfluence aphasic and that of fluent aphasic patients. Lesser also presents the use of a modified version of the test in which tokens have been replaced by concrete objects. Contrary to what one might expect, this does not make the test less sensitive, as if the use of familiar objects in an unfamiliar test situation increased its artificiality. This artificiality or perhaps, as Goldstein (1948) would say, this "abstract" aspect may well contribute quite significantly to the diagnostic power of the Token Test.

Another approach to neurolinguistic aspects of comprehension is to perform a taxonomic analysis of the Token Test in its original form, as illustrated in the chapter by Whitaker and Whitaker. They show that the Token Test commands are both linguistically complex and linguistically diverse. These factors are probably important determinants of the ability of the Token Test to detect widely different types of aphasia.

The instructions of the Token Test are ordinarily given orally. Poeck and Hartje address the question of whether a different mode of presentation (visual, in this case) modified Token Test performance by aphasic subjects. They find that when the instructions are read by the patients, their performance is comparable to that found in the ordinary, auditory presentation. These results indicate that poor Token Test results are not due merely to impaired processing of auditory signals but also are due to a disorder in the "central language system" (Whitaker, 1971).

In addition to its use in the detection of subtle deficits in auditory comprehension, the Token Test has been used to investigate other aspects of auditory behavior. These "nondiagnostic" uses are reviewed by Holland and Whitney and include studies where the test has provided information on the importance of auditory processing, speed of presentation, and experimenter's behavior during item presentation.

A different aspect of Token Test performance is explored by Noll and Lass, who have given the test to children of different socioeconomic background. They find that economically disadvantaged children perform less well on the Token Test especially in younger age groups. The interpretation of these results is undboutedly complex but they point to the importance of using appropriate normative data when interpreting Token Test results.

Zaidel illustrates the contribution of the Token Test to neuropsychology in chapter 10 in which he analyzes the contribution of each cerebral hemisphere to Token Test performance. His results are based on his work with commissurotomy and hemispherectomy patients. He shows a massive and fairly stable deficit of the right hemisphere which is attributed to that hemisphere's limited short-term verbal memory and rehearsal capacity, and to the long and ordered nonredundant Token Test instructions.

Where are the neuroanatomical lesions in patients with poor Token Test performance? The CAT Scan allows a dramatically new manner of answering that question. Vignolo presents the CAT Scan correlates of Token Test performance and identifies the cortical and subcortical areas that tend to be affected in patients with severe impairment and in those with no or only very slight impairment.

Finally, in chapter 12 Dennis summarizes the present status of the Token Test and outlines possible future directions.

# 2

## The Token Test: A Sensitive Test to Detect Receptive Disturbances in Aphasics[1]

ENNIO De RENZI AND LUIGI A. VIGNOLO

A routine clinical examination of a patient with aphasia sometimes fails to reveal the slightest receptive disorders: This happens most often either in very mild sensory aphasics or in aphasics whose disturbances seem limited to a frank expressive syndrome. In such case the examiner is compelled to challenge the language comprehension of the patient with subtler tests: In so doing, however, he almost always finds himself giving tasks which involve other intellectual functions than language alone. Consequently, if the subject fails, it is hard to decide how far his errors are due to a difficulty in "decoding" the semantic structure of the message and to what extent they are simply due to a lack of the capacity of grasping its intellectual implications. A typical illustration of this ambiguity in tests of verbal comprehension is given by Head's (1926) Hand-Eye-Ear Test, which was designed expressly to get aphasics into trouble and yet turned out to be quite difficult also for a certain number of normal individuals (Goldstein, 1950), and even for some subjects of the highest intellectual level (Weisenburg and McBride, 1935). Our own experience confirms the difficulty such tasks present for organic brain

[1]Reprinted from *Brain*, 1962, *85*, 665-678, with the permission of Oxford University Press.

patients, even including those who are free from defects in the language area.

Another widely used test is Pierre Marie's Paper Test, which consists in a series of commands connected by no logical link, to be performed in their correct order by the patient: "Here are three papers, a big one, a middle-sized one, and a little one. Take the biggest and rumple it up and throw it on the ground. Give me the middle-sized one. Put the smallest one in your pocket." This test deserves the popularity which it enjoys, for two reasons—one practical and one theoretical—which will repay further attention and should be borne in mind in designing any set of tests of receptive processes in aphasics. The practical reason, at first sight trivial, in fact reflects a principle of considerable importance: It is that Marie's test does not require any special equipment and can be applied at any moment at the patient's bedside. The theoretical reason is that its difficulty lies entirely on a linguistic level and not on an intellectual level. The orders are, in fact, extremely elementary from a conceptual standpoint and they would prove very easy even to a child. However, their comprehension is made hard by the fact that they refer to objects—the three papers—of the same nature, which can be identified only through the quantitative relations that exist between them: "big," "middle-sized," "little." From the linguistic standpoint this means that the three objects are not denoted by three clear-cut and simple semantic entities, as they would be if a separate concrete noun applied to each, but, on the contrary, by words representing a much subtler distinction, namely different degrees of the attribute "size." From this point of view the alternative test proposed by Pierre Marie himself is not as good: "Stand up, knock three times on the window with your fingers, come back in front of the table, turn once around the chair and sit down." It is clear that here the operations which the subject is required to perform involve simpler discriminations among more tangible features of the environment and, consequently, simpler and more definite linguistic denotations. This task, moreover, shows very clearly the weak point shared by both of Marie's tests, that is, the need for the patient to remember accurately a complex sequence of commands, in order to perform the tasks correctly. As a result, carelessness and confusion in the performance may sometimes be due to a defect of fixation rather than to misunderstanding, especially if aged patients are being tested.

Another test to reveal slight receptive defects is the one proposed by Thomas and Charles Roux (quoted by Ballet and Laignel-Lavastine, 1911). It consists in pronouncing before the patient a certain number of syllables, one of which forms part of the name of an object which is meanwhile shown to him. The syllable may be the first, the last, or an intermediate syllable of the given name. The patient has to recognize which syllable is the one. Such a test is undoubtedly subtle, but it requires great attention and a skill in analyzing the syllabic structure of words, i.e. in spelling words, which is not necessarily within the reach of all subjects.

Passing over various other kinds of examination—for example, Kleist's test (Kleist, 1922-1934), not very different from that of Thomas and Roux—we cannot escape mentioning the important work of Weisenburg and McBride (1935), who have systematized a conspicuous number of tests for aphasics, some of which are suited to the examination of slight receptive disorders. The book of the American Authors undoubtedly constitutes a mine of information for anyone who seeks suggestions and advice as to the examination of aphasics, although there is perhaps the risk of becoming confused among such a wealth of tests and of not knowing which are the most useful. Moreover, the most penetrating tests suggested by Weisenburg and McBride were derived from intelligence tests and their solution must therefore imply to some extent the overcoming of difficulties which are not merely verbal, but also conceptual. Language Intelligence tests such as the Opposite Test, the Part-Whole, the Analogies, the Absurdities, and so on, are quite typical in this sense. It seems clear, for example, that if we lack any other evidence (as may be the case in subclinical aphasia) we shall be in doubt how to interpret a failure to identify the absurdity included in a statement such as this: "When there is a collision, the last car of the train is usually damaged most, so the guard thinks it would be best if the last car were always taken off before the train starts." Now, this is exactly the sort of test we may be tempted to employ in cases of subclinical aphasia; yet the chances are that, in this event, we shall end up by adding more and more perplexities to our initial problems.

Finally, if it is to be clinically useful in revealing slight receptive disorders, a test must have certain qualities that can be briefly listed under the following headings:

1. The test should require only a reasonably short time.
2. It should require neither special apparatus nor specific printed material, for often neither will be available when needed.
3. It should be made up of orders so short as to be easily memorized by any normal adult, regardless of his age.
4. It should include the least possible difficulty on an intellectual level, so that any individual may be able to perform the tasks correctly, independently—within reasonable limits—of his I.Q.
5. It should contain, on the contrary, considerable difficulties on a linguistic level.

At this point, we must define more accurately what we mean by the phrase "difficulties on a linguistic level." It must first of all be realized that we do not refer to the use of unusual words and syntactic forms, since the comprehension of these depends mainly upon previous experience and the ability of the subject to profit by it; hence an intellectual or "culture" factor is involved. The difficulty must lie, on the contrary, in the lack of redundancy of the message transmitted to the patient and in the necessity, which this entails, of grasping its significance from the semantic value of every single word he hears. Lack of redundancy to this extent rarely occurs in everyday conversation, where the comprehension of speech is aided by a whole series of factors—some linguistic and some extralinguistic—which contribute towards orienting the expectancy set of the hearer in a given direction, so that he merely needs to understand some elements of the question in order to respond with an adequate answer. These contributory clues to the understanding of speech could be classified as follows:

1. Clues coming from the *situation* in which the patient finds himself and from the relation that traditionally binds him to the person he communicates with. If such a person is a physician, the patient will expect to be asked certain particular questions—questions, that is, that are usually asked during a medical examination. As Ombredane (1951) rightly points out, comprehension of a command such as "Put out your tongue" is made easier by the fact that this is a usual request when it comes from a doctor. No wonder, therefore, that it may be understood perfectly well by severe aphasics, who are unable to grasp the meaning of other equally simple but not so obvious orders.

2. Clues given the the *nature of the objects* with which the patient is invited to perform. Such clues exist when the order represents the most usual way of dealing with the object. If I put a pencil before a patient, the operations I can require him to perform are quite narrowly limited: I can tell him to write, to draw, to take the pencil, to hand it to somebody; but he can virtually ignore the possibility that I shall tell him to eat it, to light it or to tie a knot in it, requests which would rightly be more expected if he had before him, respectively, an apple, a cigarette or a piece of string.

It should be noted also that the comprehension of orders concerning an object lying in front of the patient is made easier by the very fact that such an object *is there*. In this connection we might recall a test suggested by Luria (1959), in which the examiner invites the patient to pick up various objects one by one from a selection of objects he has before him, and from time to time gives the trick-command to take up an object which is not there.

3. Clues given by the *verbal context*. Words in proposition are not uttered at random, but each of them calls for other words, according to rules determined by linguistic laws and by the nature of things. When the hearer has grasped some elements of a proposition, he can often fill in the blanks with some confidence, by referring to the words that come before and after those he has failed to understand. As Miller (1956) points out, "if one perceives enough of speech, to discover the fundamental set-up of the phrase, the number of words that can be replaced (in the perceptive blank) is much reduced; therefore, the possibility arises of making an exact guess. For example, in the statement "he threw ... out of the window," we can immediately reject all nouns which connote objects that one cannot throw. Then, we can give our preferences to objects which people use to throw, such as balls, stones, bombs and so on. So we come to a very limited number of possibilities."

Moreover, when we talk, we use many words, circumlocutions and turns of phrase which are not strictly necessary to the communication of our thought and which serve mainly to embellish its expression, to add emphasis or superfluous precision, to make it clearer or more interesting to the hearer, and which are therefore redundant as far as the essential of our communication is concerned. Consider, for instance, one of the items of a test for aphasia currently used in our clinic (De Renzi, 1960). The patient is asked the following question: "Could you tell me the name of the animal the farmer milks every day in the stable?" It is obvious that this sentence—uttered, as it is, with a questioning note—could be cut down to "the animal the farmer milks in the stable." Probably even the fragment "animal farmer milks" would suffice for the understanding of the entire question. In Marie's test, quoted above: "Stand up, knock three times on the window with your fingers, come back in front of the table, turn once around the chair and sit down," the fragments "stand up" and "come back in front of the table" are, strictly speaking, redundant, because both actions are already implied by the orders that come next.

The foregoing considerations suggest a way in which to enhance the sensitivity of a test for inapparent receptive disorders. At the level of the relation between examiner and patient no facilitation problem arises, provided that the typical requests of a medical examination are avoided. At the level of the characteristics of the material with which we will examine the patient, we can choose between two alternative courses. We can, for example, modify the operations for which the objects are habitually used, going as far as to switch the habitual use of an object with that of another. If a pencil and a toothbrush are on the table, we may ask the subject to draw a square with the toothbrush and to brush his teeth with the pencil. Alternatively, we can choose objects that are poorly differentiated, both in reality and in language, such as pieces of paper of various shapes, going on the principle that the concept, and therefore the verbal expression, "piece of paper" is far less specific than "toothbrush."

Finally, at the third level—that of verbal context—every effort must be made to give commands in a nonredundant form, that is to say, in such a way that the understanding of every single word of the sentence becomes indispensable to the right performance of the order. It must be made impossible for the hearer to deduce or to reconstruct any word he may miss by following the clues contained in the words which precede or follow it.

## THE TOKEN TEST

We hope to make some contributions to the semeiology of receptive language functions by putting forward a test based on the above-mentioned principles. The material of the test consists of tokens like those used in card games. As far as shape is concerned, there are two types of token: circles and rectangles. As far as size is concerned, there are also two types: the large ones and the small ones. Finally, there are five types of token as far as color is concerned: red, blue, green, yellow and white. Summing up, we have four rows of five tokens each: large circles, small circles, large rectangles and small rectangles; and in each row we have a red, a blue, a green, a yellow and a white token (see Figure 2.1). The peculiar characteristic of the test material is that, when all the 20 tokens are present, it is not enough to use a single word in order to identify a particular token but, on the contrary, at least three specific words are required, namely a noun and two adjectives. Thus, we will have to say, for example: "the large red rectangle," "the small red circle," and so on. If, however, large tokens only are used, two specific words—a noun and a color adjective, will suffice to identify a particular token, for we can then say merely: "the white circle," "the green rectangle," and so on. None of the specific qualifying words is redundant, that is to say, each of them must be decoded correctly in order to choose the right token. Moreover, if only two out of the three elements of the connotation are understood, they do not give any clue concerning the third element: when I am told that I must take the large rectangle I still have no clue whatsoever as to which of the large rectangles—the red, the blue, the green, etc.—the order is about. Finally, the fact that the material is constituted by tokens and not, for example, by cigarettes or pencils is

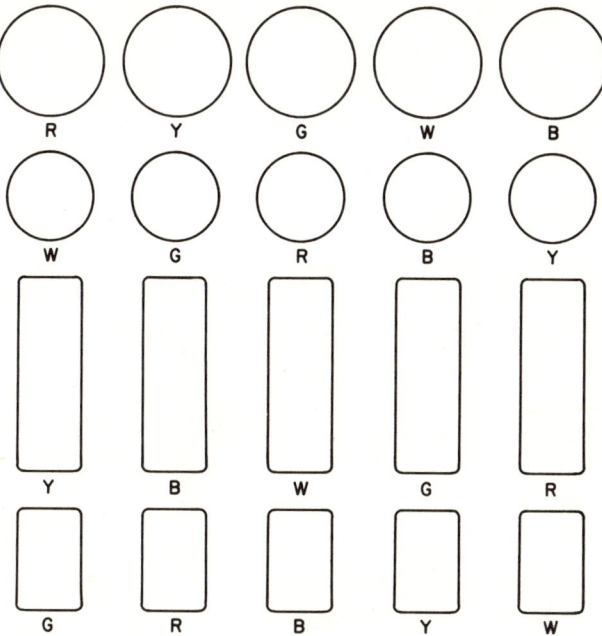

**FIGURE 2.1.** *Materials used in the Token Test. R = red, B = blue, G = green, Y = yellow, W = white. Colors are distributed entirely at random.*

quite important. Tokens, like pieces of paper, are objects that can be denoted by an abstract noun, such as "circle" and "rectangle." We will come back to this point later, when we will come to discuss the results of the test.

The test is built up of five parts, progressively more and more difficult. In the first four parts, commands are expressed in an elementary grammatical and syntactic form: verb, object. In the fifth part we have tried to make the test more difficult by introducing grammatical particles or other more complex syntactic structures, the exact understanding of which is always necessary to a correct performance. Before starting one must make sure that the patient has no agnosic disturbances as far as form and color recognition is concerned and understands the meaning of the words "circle" and "rectangle" and of the five colors to be eventually called forth.

*First part.*—Large rectangles and large circles only are arranged on the table in two rows. There is no particular rule for the distribution of colors. Speaking with a clear and measured voice, without any special prosodic emphasis, the examiner invites the patient to take ten different tokens, one after the other, saying simply: "Pick up the yellow rectangle," "Pick up the white circle," and so on. The patient must put back each token in its place on each occasion.

*Second part.*—Small circles and small rectangles are added to the tokens already on the table, in the arrangement shown in Figure 2.1. Three specific words are now necessary in order to identify a particular token. Ten commands are given, of the type: "Pick up the small white rectangle," "Pick up the large blue circle," and so on.

*Third part.*—Large tokens only are placed before the subject, as in the first part: here, however, the patient is invited to take two of them, for example: "Take the red circle and the green rectangle." Ten commands are given, connoting 20 different tokens.

*Fourth part.*—All tokens are on the table again, as in the second part, and the patient is asked to take two of them every time: "Take the white large circle and the small green rectangle." Ten performances are required.

*Fifth part.*—Large rectangles are put in the first row before the patient and large circles are put in the second row. There is no particular rule for the distribution of colors, except that the yellow rectangle must be near the green one, so as to allow item 7 to be applied. Orders are as follows:

1. Put the red circle on the green rectangle.
2. Put the white rectangle behind the yellow circle.
3. Touch the blue circle with the red rectangle.
4. Touch—with the blue circle—the red rectangle.
5. Touch the blue circle and the red rectangle.
6. Pick up the blue circle or the red rectangle.
7. Put the green rectangle away from the yellow rectangle.
8. Put the white circle before the blue rectangle.
9. If there is a black circle, pick up the red rectangle.

*N. B. There is no black circle.*
10. Pick up the rectangles, except the yellow one.
11. When I touch the green circle, you take the white rectangle.

*N. B. Wait a few seconds before touching the green circle.*
12. Put the green rectangle beside the red circle.
13. Touch the rectangles, slowly, and the circles, quickly.
14. Put the red circle between the yellow rectangle and the green rectangle.
15. Except for the green one, touch the circles.
16. Pick up the red circle—no!—the white rectangle.
17. Instead of the white rectangle, take the yellow circle.

18. Together with the yellow circle, take the blue circle.
19. After picking up the green rectangle, touch the white circle.
20. Put the blue circle under the white rectangle.
21. Before touching the yellow circle, pick up the red rectangle.

As one can see, this last part is quite different from the others. In the former four parts, in fact, orders comprised only a verb (always the same) and an object, so that the attention of the patient was allowed to concentrate entirely on the task of identifying the latter element of the order. On the contrary, most of the statements of the fifth part include a new grammatical element, i.e. a preposition, a conjunction or an adverb. These are small enough additions to the message, as far as its length is concerned, but they suffice to give the message a much greater linguistic subtlety and to change radically the meaning of the action that the patient is required to perform. Now it is not enough to understand the isolated meaning of the new particle, but it is also necessary to grasp its contextual meaning, i.e., to determine to which other element of the sentence it refers. In some cases it is essential to pay attention to the position that such a grammatical element occupies within the sentence, since a small displacement is sufficient to reverse the meaning of the command. This is illustrated by the two following items: "Touch the blue circle with the red rectangle" and "Touch—with the blue circle—the red rectangle."

A particular emphasis has been put on prepositions denoting spatial relations between objects, for these are quite difficult for aphasics to understand, as Ombredane has shown by his Cat and Chair Test. The same prepositions are usually understood by patients with spatial agnosia, except for the terms "right" and "left," which have not been included in our test for this reason. A special remark should be made about the prepositions "before" and "behind." A normal subject dealing with the tokens arranged in the forementioned order on the table may interpret "before" as connoting either a position "nearer to" himself or a position "farther from" himself. This possibility should be remembered during the examination, and it is advisable that the examiner wait until both items 2 and 8 are performed before scoring them.

A small group of 4 statements—items 9, 12, 20, 22—include a subordinate clause, that modifies, limits or suspends the command expressed in the main clause. Here the subject, in order to understand well, must keep in mind both principal and subordinate information until the message is over, so as to be able to put them in their adequate reciprocal relation and treat the command as a whole. Consider, for example, item 9: "If there is a black circle, pick up the red rectangle."

The meaning of the main clause "Pick up the red rectangle" is completely altered by the condition introduced by the subordinate clause "If there is a black circle," for, as there is no black circle, the meaning of the order turns out to be: "Do *not* take the red rectangle."

Summing up, here we have a number of messages, sufficiently elementary from a conceptual standpoint, short and easy to memorize (the longest of them contains 19 syllables against the 48 syllables of Pierre Marie's test), which, however, make two kinds of demand upon the comprehension of the patient: One arises out of the difficulty of identifying a particular token specified by three independent features and the other from that of grasping the semantic complications introduced by the "small instruments of language."[2]

## RESULTS

All aphasics who, at a normal clinical examination of aphasia, already show clear disturbances in the understanding of speech have serious difficulty in the performance of the Token Test. The test, however, is not made for them, but rather for those aphasic patients in whom receptive disorders seem very slight or altogether lacking during normal conversation: They are mild sensory aphasics, or motor aphasics with a defect apparently confined to the expressive side.

Among this latter type of patients we have selected 13 "pure" motor aphasics—at least 5 of which could be classified as cases of "anarthrie" as defined by the French Authors—and 6 sensory aphasics at a stage of very good regression of the symptoms: None of them showed any difficulty of understanding during a normal conversation. Each of these patients had been examined also with a complete test for aphasia used in our clinic (De Renzi, 1960), and most of them had no receptive difficulty throughout all the 54 items of that battery. Thus, their language comprehension appeared to be unimpaired despite an investigation far more thorough than a routine clinical examination of aphasia.

In each of these cases, the Token Test has revealed clear disturbances in the understanding of oral messages. As would be expected, the

---

[2] It should be noted that the test has been originally designed for and applied to Italian patients. The orders presented here are the same, translated into English as accurately as possible: Therefore, they should be considered merely as a demonstration of the degree of difficulty of the different items. It would be convenient, perhaps, to substitute or modify some of them, so as to make them convey, in English, differences of meaning comparable to those involved in the original Italian text.

mildest aphasics perform the first part quite well, and often even the second and third part—although some errors may appear quite unexpectedly here and there—but in the fourth and fifth part mistakes become very frequent. We will deal later more broadly on the nature of such mistakes. Here it is the following case of presenile cerebral atrophy, which, we think, deserves the qualification of latent aphasia, at least in the sense that, on the clinical level, none of the neurologists who had previously examined him had suspected the presence of language disturbances. The patient was a 60-year-old mechanical engineer, who had been suffering for six months from a conspicuous reduction of his working capacities and from memory defects. The neurological and general medical examination showed no evidence of disease. The psychological examination, on the contrary, revealed a certain mental deterioration, with lowered associative power, poor capacity for original judgment, amnesia for recent facts, disturbances in calculation and apathy with some tendency towards depression. At the Wechsler test he had a I.Q. = 92, with, however, a M.D. = 66 per cent; at the vocabulary subtest he obtained a high score: 13. At the Weigl test he succeeded in classifying only according to color. The pneumoencephalography showed a conspicuous dilatation of both lateral ventricles, especially of their temporal horns, without displacement. The cerebro-spinal fluid was normal. The patient seemed to understand everything he was told and expressed himself correctly from a linguistic standpoint. Reading and writing were good. At the Token Test, he started making a great number of mistakes in the second and third part, and ended up with gross and frequent errors in the fourth and fifth part. Such mistakes were not due to a fixation memory defect, because the patient repeated the order to himself correctly aloud and yet performed it wrongly, thereby showing that he had grossly misunderstood its meaning. We tried to check the presence of aphasia with further examinations: Among the Weisenburg and McBride battery of tests, the patient did well in the Sentence Completion, both Oral and Printed—except for one slight perseveration. Opposites were easily identified. Oral Analogies and Oral Absurdities gave him considerable trouble. He had a very hard time in building up sentences with three given words (from Terman's Test), and he often failed altogether. The best evidence of aphasia was provided, however, by his poor performance in Ombredane's tests, that is the Cat and Chair Test and Caran D'Ache's cartoons.

In this, as in the other cases where the test has been applied, one could object that mistakes depend more on a general intellectual defect than on true aphasia. From a theoretical standpoint, such an hypothesis seems rather improbable, since, as we have already said, the orders employed are conceptually very simple and do not involve any unusual or odd linguistic form. On experimental grounds, moreover, we have observed that the test is performed quite well even by non-aphasic subjects with intellectual deterioration, provided that their mental condition leaves them a certain capacity for concentration. Finally, at least three of the patients with anarthrie who have shown poor comprehension in this test perform well in non-linguistic tests.

It might be interesting to try to analyse qualitatively the types of mistake most frequently encountered. One could discover, for example, whether certain linguistic elements appear to be recognized worse than others by aphasics. This kind of analysis is quite simple so far as parts one to four are concerned. In order to make classification easier, it will be convenient to represent by capital letters the various parts of the message and to underline the letter corresponding to the part which has been misunderstood. For example, the statement "Take the small white circle" can be outlined thus: V (verb)—A'(size adjective)—A"(color adjective)—N(noun). If the patient takes the small white rectangle instead of the small white circle, we will write: V—A'—A"—N, underlining the N. The verb is always identical and therefore it may be overlooked.

It should be noted that if the subject were to choose entirely at random he would have a 50 per cent chance of guessing the right noun and the right size adjective—but he would have only a 20 per cent chance of guessing the right color adjective, since 5 colors occur in the test. Even leaving aside this aspect of the problem, we must consider that nouns are presented 60 times during the first 4 parts of the test, while adjectives are presented 90 times. This means that we should expect the greatest number of errors to fall within adjectives in general, and color adjectives in particular. On the contrary, the total count of errors reveals that—speaking in absolute figures—they affect nouns more often than adjectives. In fact, in parts one to four, the performances of all the patients submitted to the test show 152 errors due to misunderstanding of nouns versus 104 errors due to misunderstanding of adjectives. One might jump to the conclusion that nouns represent a weaker category than adjectives, but we think that such an hypothesis, tempting as it may be, must be discarded, and that the unequal distribution of errors must be attributed to the peculiar type of noun employed in the test. In fact, by applying to the same patients another version of the test, where several objects, like pencils, thimbles, toothbrushes and so on, of five different colors, are used instead of tokens, we have noticed that the understanding of nouns was far less affected than that of adjectives.[3] The reason for

---

[3]Incidentally, we must say that the test, thus modified, is definitely less sensitive.

this fact is that there is, we think, an important difference between a noun such as "pencil" and a noun such as "circle" or "rectangle," as employed in the test: the former is indissolubly bound to a very specific object, which it denotes in its whole, indivisible unity, while the latter identifies an attribute of the token—its form—like the adjective "red" identifies its color and "large" its size. In this sense, "circle" and "rectangle" are really adjectives pretending—so to speak—to be nouns. If such an equivalence between the nouns denoting form and the adjectives denoting color and size is true, then the purely formal distinction noun versus adjective seems senseless here and should be substituted by the distinction between "verbal expressions denoting form," "verbal expressions denoting color" and "verbal expressions denoting size." The results of the test reveal that verbal expressions denoting form are understood worse than the others. A tentative explanation for this fact could be that shape is possibly a more abstract concept than color or size, geometrical conceptions—and their linguistic equivalents—being learned later than size and color-discrimination in childhood.

In the fifth part of the test, as we have said above, other grammatical elements—prepositions, conjunctions, adverbs—have been introduced; and it would be interesting to know whether aphasics find it more difficult to grasp the meaning of such elements than that of the "nouns" and adjectives which appear in the same commands. It must be pointed out however, that the test, in its present form, has not been designed specifically to answer this question. Furthermore, it has not been applied to a sufficiently large number of cases to afford us any firm conclusion. What follows is, therefore, no more than a hint for future research.

In every item of part five, expressions denoting form, color, and size ("nouns" and adjectives) on the one side, and grammatical particles on the other are unequally represented. In fact, there are two "nouns," two adjectives and one particle in almost every item. Consequently, if mistakes were determined by mere chance, they should fall on the group of the expressions denoting form, color, and size more often than they would on the particles, according to a four-to-one ratio. On the contrary, we find 120 errors on particles versus 101 errors on "nouns" and adjectives: This means that wrong performances are due a little more often to misunderstanding of the particle. Some of them appear particularly weak: They are spacial prepositions such as "on," "under," "before," "behind," the disjunctive particle "or," the contradictory "—no!—," the conditional "if." However, while it seems sensible to us to believe that grammatical particles are impaired in aphasia more easily than expressions denoting form, color and size—because they have a merely connecting function, because they have no semantic independence, and finally because they have been acquired late in the development of language—we do not feel able to determine which of them are more impaired and which are less impaired on the basis of the present results. It is hard to see how prepositions, conjunctions, and adverbs could be evaluated in terms of their abstract difficulty. It seems, rather, that they must be considered within a given context, and it must be admitted that contexts are not the same throughout the Token Test: Commands differ from each other in respects both structural and conceptual. For example, an order such as "Instead of the white rectangle, take the yellow circle" is probably easier than the conceptually similar "Take the red circle—no!—the white rectangle," because in the first case the adverb is put at the beginning of the order and therefore raises the expectation of a correcting message to come, whereas in the second case it shows up after the order has been given, cancels it quite unexpectedly and compels the hearer to switch his attention towards a completely different task. On the other hand, the order "If there is a black circle, take the red rectangle" contains a little conceptual trick: For the first time during the test, a command refers to an object which is not on the table, and coming, as it does, after so many positive orders, it ends up inviting the patient to do nothing at all. This overall experimental context, rather than the use of a conditional clause, may be responsible for the difficulty of the item.

At all events, it seems to us that the Token Test, if analyzed from this viewpoint, might provide some interesting data for that linguistic approach to aphasia which many contemporary authors consider to be promising and from which Wepman *et al.* (1956) and Goodglass and Hunt (1958) have already obtained fruitful results.

The Token Test, however, must be considered above all as a practical clinical tool, endowed of great sensitivity and contaminated as little as possible by intellectual difficulties.

## SUMMARY

After having discussed the characteristics that an examination of the receptive language processes in aphasics should have in order to reveal slight disturbances in the understanding of speech, without challenging other intellectual functions than language alone, the authors describe a test designed to that purpose. Tokens of 2 different shapes, 2 different sizes, and 5 different colors are arranged on the table in front of the patient, who is then given oral commands expressed in progressively more and more complex, non-redundant messages. In response to these orders, the patient must perform very simple manual tasks with the tokens, such as picking up, touching or moving one or several of them. The sensitivity of the test seems proved by the fact that it revealed clear disturbances of speech comprehension in each of the 19 patients submitted to it—13 "pure" motor aphasics and 6 sensory aphasics at an advanced stage of recovery, none of whom had ever shown any difficulty in understanding during a normal conversation. Finally, the authors suggest some tentative explanations of the types of mistakes more frequently encountered, based on the analysis of the linguistic elements more easily affected by the receptive disorder.

## ACKNOWLEDGMENT

The authors wish to thank Dr. Hugh Thomas for his helpful suggestions in reading the English text.

# II
## REVISED TESTS

# 3
## A Shortened Version of the Token Test[1]

ENNIO DE RENZI

In 1962, De Renzi and Vignolo proposed the Token Test as a means of revealing mild disturbances of verbal comprehension in aphasics. According to the authors, the advantages of this test over other tests of comprehension (e.g., the Paper Test of Pierre Marie; the Eye–Nose–Ear Test of Head; the Cat and Chair Test of Ombredane; the many tests of verbal intelligence used by Weisenburg and McBride) may be summarized as follows:

1. Use of material with elementary perceptual characteristics (20 round and rectangular tokens of five different colors and two different sizes) to avoid problems of visual recognition, especially in patients with lesions of the posterior areas of the brain.
2. Commands that are brief, simple in lexical and syntactic structure, and possessing minimal intellectual demands. Comprehension may therefore be expected to be independent of the patient's educational background, level of intelligence, and, to a certain extent, of his short-term verbal memory capacity.
3. Difficulty of individual items residing essentially in low verbal redundancy of the message. Reconstruction of the command cannot be made on the basis of context. This means that the

[1]This work was supported by a grant from the Consiglio Nazionale delle Richerche.

patient must decode every element of the command in order to respond correctly. For example, the command "Touch the *small yellow circle*" involves comprehension of each of the three words; having understood two of them (*circle, small*) does not help in any way in reconstructing the third (*yellow*).

In the original study, De Renzi and Vignolo (1962) presented data showing poor performance on this test by 13 aphasics chosen for their lack of demonstrable comprehension disturbances on clinical examination. A more systematic study was executed by Boller and Vignolo (1966), who administered the test to normal subjects, patients with right hemisphere lesions, nonaphasic left hemisphere patients, and left hemisphere aphasics with language disturbances apparently confined to expression. Taking as cut-off point the worst score obtained by a normal subject, 87% of motor aphasics, 35% of left hemisphere patients judged not to be aphasic, but only one of 30 right brain-damaged patients performed at a significantly low level on the Token Test. The authors drew the inference that the test is not sensitive to cerebral damage in general, but to lesions of the areas subserving language ability.

Simplicity of administration and diagnostic sensitivity have won for the Token Test considerable popularity among students of aphasia: It has been the subject of experimentation in Germany (Orgass & Poeck, 1966, 1969; Poeck, Kerschensteiner, & Hartje, 1972; Poeck, Orgass, Kerschensteiner, & Hartje, 1974; Hartje, Kerschensteiner, Poeck, & Orgass, 1973; Sipos and Tägert, 1972; Orgass, 1975; Tägert, Chock, Niklas, Sandvoss, & Sipos, 1975), in England (Lesser, 1974), in the United States (Swisher & Sarno, 1969), in Romania (Kreindler, Gheorghita, & Voirescu, 1971), in Finland (Vilkki & Laitinen, 1974), and in Italy (Boller, 1968; Parisi & Pizzamiglio, 1970; Pizzamiglio & Appicciafuoco, 1971). Yet, the clinical use of the test has been to a certain extent hindered by lack of precise normative data, providing criteria for differentiating a normal from a pathological performance. This circumstance encouraged a rather loose use of the test: Some authors considerably reduced the number of items; others changed the scoring system; still others varied the shape and colors of the tokens. Although the changes the test has undergone have not detracted from its popularity as an effective tool to diagnose aphasia, and may have even enlarged the scope of its application, they have left the scientific community without a conventional form of the test to which everybody may refer when discussing results obtained in different groups of patients.

It has also been apparent, since the early investigations, that the test could be reduced in length without substantial loss of information. The original version of the test provided for four parts of 10 items each, having the form verb + object complement, and involving the comprehension of two, three, four, and six words, respectively; for example, "Touch the *red circle*," "Touch the *large green rectangle*," "Touch the *yellow circle* and the *white rectangle*," "Touch the *small red circle* and the *large yellow circle*." There was also a fifth part consisting of 21 items of more complex syntactic structure. In these 21 items, the decoding of grammatical particles (prepositions, conjunctions, adverbs) is necessary for accurate comprehension of the command: for example, *"Put the green rectangle next to the red circle."* Spellacy and Spreen (1969) showed that it was possible to reduce the original 61 items of the test to 16 while still maintaining good reliability and discriminative capacity.

For many years, we have been using an abbreviated form of the Token Test and have given it to a large number of subjects free from cerebral damage, both children and adults, as well as to brain-damaged patients with and without aphasia. The number of test items has been reduced, and a new section (Section 1) introduced containing 7 minimally difficult items which require comprehension of only one word, for example, "Touch a *circle*." This was done to broaden the diagnostic capacity of the test for aphasics with severe comprehension deficit, whose comprehension score would otherwise be zero.

Other modifications have been introduced in the materials of the test. The first change, substitution of squares for rectangles, was suggested by the greater frequency of occurrence of the former word (considering its use as both a substantive and an adjective) in comparison with the latter (Bortolini, Tagliavini, & Zampoli, 1972). The second modification consists of substituting black tokens for blue ones. It has been demonstrated that both brain-damaged patients and normal adults show a certain degree of difficulty in discriminating blue and green (Scotti & Spinnler, 1970). Since there were both blue and green tokens in the test, we wished to avoid an undesirable factor of color confusion.

The present report summarizes the results obtained administering the new version of the Token Test to large numbers of normal controls and brain-damaged patients (De Renzi & Faglioni, 1975, 1978).

## THE TOKEN TEST

The test consists of 20 plastic tokens 3 mm in thickness. There are 10 *circles* and 10 *squares*. Five circles and squares are *large,* that is, 30 mm on each side or in diameter, respectively, and 5 circles and squares are *small,* that is, 20 mm on each side or in diameter, respectively. In each series of 5 circles or squares, the following colors are represented: *black, white, red, yellow* and *green*. When all 20 tokens are used, their arrangement on the table is that indicated in Figure 3.1.

The patient is seated in front of the token array and is told "As you see, there are 20 tokens here. Some of them are squares [the experimenter quickly puts his finger on the two series of squares], while others are circles [he does the same]. Some are large, others are small [he so indicates]. There are red ones, black, green, yellow and white ones [each time he points to the tokens of the color named]. Now, I'm going to tell you to touch one of these tokens: Touch a circle." If the subject asks, "Which one?", the experimenter answers, "Whichever one you want: Just touch a circle." In giving the commands the words should be uttered distinctly and without any special prosodic emphasis, with the exception of the "no" in item 34, which is accentuated and followed by a brief pause, before saying "the white squares." The test items appear in the appendix. If, following each command of Parts 1–5, the patient fails to initiate a response after 5 sec, or if he responds incorrectly, the examiner returns the tokens to their original order and says "Let's try that again," and then repeats the command. One point is credited for a correct

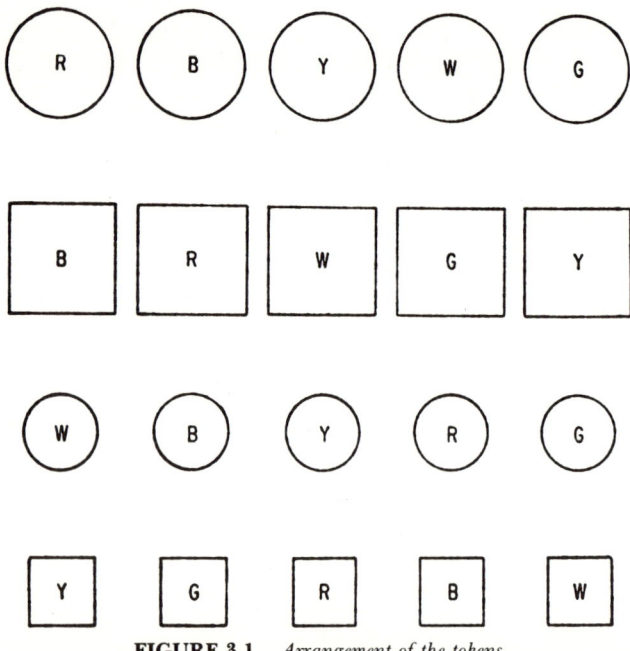

**FIGURE 3.1.** *Arrangement of the tokens.*

performance on the first presentation and .5 point if the performance is correct only on the second presentation. The global scores are rounded to the upper figure. The items of the sixth part are not repeated, because experience has shown that patients usually do not benefit from a second presentation and often become frustrated. Corrections made spontaneously are accepted. If the patient complains that he has forgotten part of the command, he is told that he should do as much as he remembers. If no correct response occurs in five successive items of the first five parts, the test is discontinued. However, Part 6 is given in its entirety, whenever the performance of the patient on the earlier parts makes him eligible to take it.

*Subjects*

Only right-handed subjects were tested. The *control group* consisted of 215 subjects, a majority admitted to the wards for disease involving the spinal cord, peripheral nerves, muscles or else eventually diagnosed free from cerebral pathology; a minority consisting of relatives of inpatients, nurses, or acquaintances of the investigators. The *aphasic group* was made up of 200 patients with injury to the left hemisphere, who had been examined in the course of several years and who proved to be impaired on one or more subsections of a standard aphasia battery. No special attempt was made to select patients in the aphasic group according to predetermined criteria; in general, they may be considered representative of the aphasia population in the setting of a neurological department. Cerebrovascular accidents were the most common etiology, followed by neoplasm, trauma, and cerebral atrophy. The time elapsed since onset of aphasia ranged from 1 day to 12 years. The *left brain-damaged nonaphasic group* consisted of 50 patients for whom there was evidence that the cerebral damage was confined to the left hemisphere, but who did not show signs of language impairment on either clinical examination or the standard aphasia battery. The *right brain-damaged group* was made up of 130 patients, whose disease was diagnosed as involving the right hemisphere only. The incidence of different etiologies in these two groups was similar to that found in the aphasic patients.

*Results*

CONTROL GROUP

Table 3.1 shows the distribution of the normal subjects' scores. The first step was to assess the influence of age and educational level on

**TABLE 3.1**
*Distribution of Normal Subjects' Scores*

|  | Number of subjects | |
|---|---|---|
| Token Test scores | Raw scores | Adjusted scores |
| 36 | 21 | 14 |
| 35 | 35 | 34 |
| 34 | 43 | 33 |
| 33 | 33 | 56 |
| 32 | 29 | 36 |
| 31 | 21 | 22 |
| 30 | 18 | 7 |
| 29 | 5 | 2 |
| 28 | 2 | 6 |
| 27 | 3 | 2 |
| 26 | 2 | – |
| 25 | – | 1 |
| 24 | 1 | – |
| 23 | – | 1 |
| 22 | 1 | 1 |
| 21 | 1 | – |

performance by computing the regression coefficients of the test scores on these two factors. In keeping with Orgass and Poeck's (1966) findings, the effect of age was negligible, $r = -.03$. The effect of years of schooling was more substantial, $r = .30$ ($p < .001$, $df = 213$). To partial out its influence on the performance, the normal subjects' scores were corrected according to the formula: (observed score + 2.36) $-.3$ (years of schooling). This procedure was also effective in normalizing the score distribution. The mean of the adjusted scores was 32.86 ($SD = 2.14$). The cut-off score distinguishing a normal from a pathological performance was determined by computing the 90% tolerance interval around the mean (Lieberman & Miller, 1963): The score of 29 corresponded to the lower tolerance limit, below which 5% of the normal population is expected to fail. In our sample 11 subjects had an adjusted score less than 29, which corresponds exactly to 5%. An expeditious way to transform observed scores into adjusted scores is to add 1 point for subjects with 3–6 years of schooling, and to subtract 1 point for subjects with 10–12 years of schooling, 2 points for subjects with 13–16 years of schooling, and 3 points for subjects with 17 years of schooling.

APHASIC GROUP

The scores of aphasic patients were extremely dispersed, ranging from 0 to 33 points. They were corrected for years of schooling by the same formula used for normals. The adjusted scores have a mean of 17.05 ($SD$ = 7.81). Fourteen patients (7%) attained or exceeded the cut-off score of 29.

The sensitivity of the Token Test in detecting impairment of oral comprehension may be better appreciated by comparing the percentage of wrong classifications with that obtained administering to the same patients a 10-phrase comprehension test, which is used in our Aphasia Standard Examination. It is composed of the following commands:

1. Open the book.
2. Blow your nose.
3. Raise your left hand.
4. Give me the ashtray.
5. Put the pencil in your pocket.
6. Knock on the table.
7. Fold the sheet in four.
8. Touch your forehead.
9. Turn over the wastebasket.
10. Look at the mirror.

Each item can be repeated a second time; the patient receives 1 point if the item is correctly executed immediately and .5 point if it is correctly executed only on the second presentation. On the basis of the performance of 50 normal subjects, the cut-off score at the 5% level, has been set at 8.5 points. The data of the phrase comprehension test were available for 106 out of 200 aphasics. Forty-two (40%) scored above the cut-off point, while the corresponding number for the Token Test was 8 (7.5%).

It has been maintained (Cohen, Kelter, Engel, Lis, & Strohner, 1976; Orgass & Poeck, 1966), that the Token Test does not discriminate between fluent and nonfluent aphasics, although subsequently Poeck, Hartje, Kerschenstein, and Orgass (1973), Orgass (1975) provided evidence that sensory aphasics are more impaired than motor and amnesic aphasics. In our sample, 108 patients were diagnosed as fluent and 71 as nonfluent on the basis of their speech output in free conversation, open ended questions and a tell-a-story test [the remaining patients belonged to conduction aphasia (7) and to other less represented categories, such as pure anomia, word deafness, agraphia, alexia, and alexia plus agraphia]. The mean of the two groups were: fluent = 16.38 ($SD$ = 7.86); nonfluent = 17.02 ($SD$ = 8.04. This difference falls far short of the significance level ($t$ = .53, n.s.). One must keep in mind, however, that the heading of nonfluent aphasia encompasses two categories of patients, Broca's and global aphasics, with lesions restricted, respectively, to the pars opercularis of the third frontal convolution and adjacent region, and to the entire language area. Since the distinction between these two forms rests at the clinical level on the degree of the comprehension impairment, which is mild to moderate in Broca's aphasics and severe in global aphasics, we suggest using the Token Test mean (17) of our aphasic sample as an objective measure for distinguishing between Broca's and global aphasics. Thus, nonfluent aphasics scoring 17 or more would be considered Broca's, those scoring less than 17, global. On the same grounds, Table 3.2 proposes a classification of the comprehension deficit, which hinges on the mean score ±1 standard deviation and defines four levels of impairment. Its value is, obviously, only practical, and it simply aims at providing objective criteria for making clinical evaluation. The number of patients of our sample falling in each category is also given.

NONAPHASIC LEFT BRAIN-DAMAGED GROUP

Correcting the scores of these patients for years of schooling showed that 42 (84%) scored 29 or higher and were, therefore, correctly identified as nonaphasic. Most of those who scored below 29 did so only marginally; the lowest score was 21.

RIGHT BRAIN-DAMAGED GROUP

When the scores of the 130 right brain-damaged patients were submitted to the same correction for years of schooling adopted with control subjects, 109 of them (84%) were found to perform within the normal range, that is, at or above the score of 29. Only 10 (7%) scored below 25 (the cut-off point for a mild impairment) and among them there were 5 patients with a severe neglect for the left half of the space, which might have prevented them from scanning the whole array of tokens.

**TABLE 3.2**
*Levels of Comprehension Deficit in Aphasics According to the Token Test Scores*

| Score | Impairment | Number of patients in each group |
|---|---|---|
| 36–29 | nil | 14 ( 7%) |
| 28–25 | mild | 20 (10%) |
| 24–17 | moderate | 76 (38%) |
| 16–9 | severe | 58 (29%) |
| 8–0 | very severe | 32 (16%) |

## DISCUSSION

It has been observed (Berry, 1973) that the large number of modifications the Token Test has undergone has resulted in the lack of a single recognized form of the test: "Clinical aphasiology now has a family of Token Tests, related, but not identical twins of their ancestors [Berry, 1973]." Proliferation is always a sign of sound and strong constitution, and different formats of the test may be suited to meet the requirements of different scientific purposes, but it is undeniable that in clinical practice a standardized version to which people can refer for assessment of verbal comprehension would be highly valuable. The present 36-item form represents a compromise between the original 61-item version and that proposed by Spellacy and Spreen (1969) consisting of only 16 items. Its administration usually takes 10-15 min and the "pass-fail" method simplifies the scoring. The introduction of the first part, with items requiring the comprehension of just one word, extends the scope of the test to include patients with severe receptive impairment. The cut-off score has been determined with reference to the control subjects' performance and educational level, the effect of which is small, although not negligible. Since the size of the control sample was large, it is reasonable to think that the score distribution has been well estimated in normals. In a previous study (De Renzi & Faglioni, 1975) we attempted to determine the cut-off score using the method of the discriminant function, which appears to be, in principle, more correct. However, since the distribution curves of the normal and the aphasic scores were dissimilar, the cut-off score we obtained turned out to be strict for the normals (.9% of them were classified as aphasic) and lenient for the aphasics (15% of them were classified as normal). The proportion of incorrect diagnoses is more balanced with the method reported here, being 5% for the normals and 7% for the aphasics. The high hit rate of the Token Test is confirmed in the present research and comes out quite clearly when it is compared with that of a common sentence comprehension test, which fails to detect comprehension deficit in 40% of aphasics.

The sensitivity of the test as an indicator of aphasia is intriguing, because of the apparent simplicity of its commands and the elementary level of the linguistic knowledge it requires. This is also attested by the performance levels of children 7-11 years old, on the present version of the test. The means obtained by each age group are reported in Figure 3.2, which also provides for comparison, the mean scores of the 215 normal adults subdivided according to their years of schooling. It is apparent that the mean score of adults with 3-5 years of schooling is comparable to that of 9-year-olds (i.e., third grade children) and that

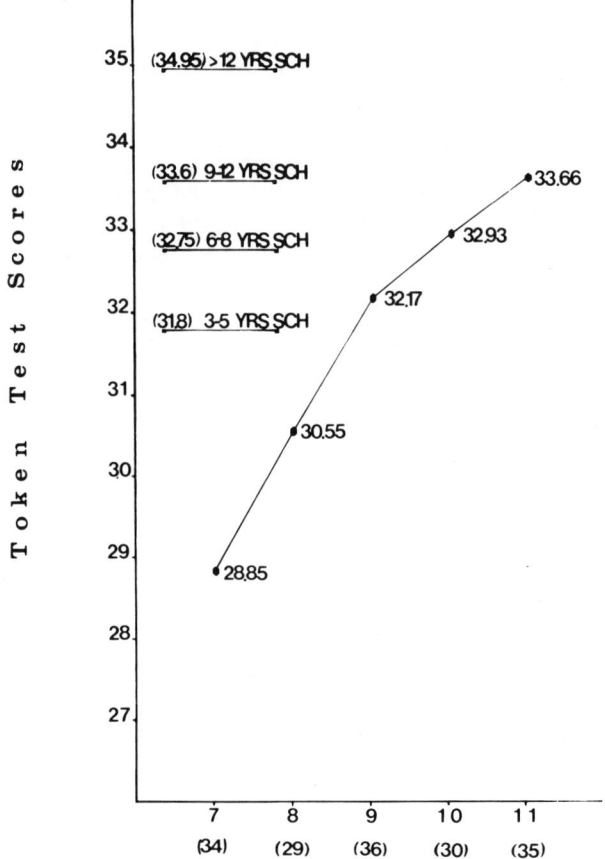

**FIGURE 3.2.** *Mean Token Test scores of children, age 7-11. The number of subjects for each age group are shown within parentheses. Horizontal lines show mean scores of normal adults subdivided by years of schooling.*

11-year-olds (i.e., fifth grade children) perform at about the same level as normal adults with 9-12 years of schooling. These data indicate that the linguistic competence needed to perform the Token Test commands is acquired early and does not entail a sophisticated mastery of language.

Consequently, the main factors contributing to the impairment of aphasic patients on the Token Test are to be found in the lack of redundancy of the message and in the absence of contextual cues, which are the unique features of the test. It ensues that the aphasics' poor performance on the test may be disproportionate to their understanding of language in real-life situations. It is in fact not rare to observe aphasic patients whose conversational comprehension appears to be adequate but who nevertheless fail dramatically on the Token Test. One should, therefore, be cautious in inferring from the Token Test performance the degree of oral comprehension impairment the patient is actually showing in everyday conditions. The discrepancy between the outcome of formal testing and the impression gained by evaluating comprehension using usual redundant messages has been recently stressed with reference to the language capability of the disconnected right hemisphere (Zaidel, 1977) and of the "wild child" Genie (Curtiss, 1977), who was claimed to have acquired speech using the right side of the brain. Following Zaidel's (1977) suggestion, the superiority of the left hemisphere in decoding nonredundant verbal information may at least in part reside in its more proficient short-term memory mechanisms, which ensure the availability for rehearsal of the single elements of the message. An increased susceptibility of the aphasics' short-term verbal memory to a distractor task has been shown by De Renzi, Faglioni, and Previdi (1978) with Token Test items and it is also remarkable that left hemisphere patients with reduced verbal memory span but good comprehension have been found impaired on the Token Test (Warrington, Logue, & Pratt, 1971).

Our findings are in agreement wit with those of previous investigators (Orgass & Poeck, 1966; Cohen *et al.*, 1976), who did not find difference in the comprehension impairment shown by fluent and nonfluent aphasics. This is not to say, however, that the Token Test fails to discriminate between anterior and posterior lesions, or between Broca's and Wernicke's aphasia, because nonfluency encompasses both patients with damage restricted to the anterior area and patients with damage of the entire language area. Our suggestion that the mean of the whole aphasic sample (17) be used to distinguish between Broca's and global aphasics rests on the assumption that a severe comprehension deficit points to a lesion encroaching upon the posterior temporal lobe, but this claim should be verified on the basis of independent anatomical or neuroradiological data. For the time being, it must be taken as a provisional mark to which one may refer when exchanging information on the language features of a given group of patients. Scores lower than 17 indicate a severe comprehension deficit, and scores lower than 9 point to the inability of the patient to understand most of verbal communication. It is worth stressing that in an unselected sample seen in a neurological department 16% of the aphasics belong to this category.

In conclusion, the present version of the Token Test aims at providing a standardized and highly sensitive tool to detect comprehension disorders in aphasics and at offering points of reference to evaluate the severity of the deficit.

## APPENDIX

Part 1. All 20 tokens displayed as in Figure 3.1.
   1. *Touch a circle.*
   2. *Touch a square.*
   3. *Touch a yellow token.*
   4. *Touch a red one.*
   5. *Touch a black one.*
   6. *Touch a green one.*
   7. *Touch a white one.*

Part 2. The small tokens are removed.
   8. *Touch the yellow square.*
   9. *Touch the black circle.*
   10. *Touch the green circle.*
   11. *Touch the white square.*

Part 3. The small tokens are replaced.
   12. *Touch the small white circle.*
   13. *Touch the large yellow square.*
   14. *Touch the large green square.*
   15. *Touch the small black circle.*

Part 4. The small tokens are removed.
   16. *Touch the red circle and the green square.*
   17. *Touch the yellow square and the black square.*
   18. *Touch the white square and the green circle.*
   19. *Touch the white circle and the red circle.*

Part 5. The small tokens are replaced.
   20. *Touch the large white circle and the small green square.*
   21. *Touch the small black circle and the large yellow square.*
   22. *Touch the large green square and the large red square.*
   23. *Touch the large white square and the small green circle.*

Part 6. The small tokens are removed.
   24. *Put the red circle on the green square.*
   25. *Touch the black circle with the red square.*
   26. *Touch the black circle and the red square.*
   27. *Touch the black circle or the red square.*
   28. *Put the green square away from the yellow square.*
   29. *If there is a blue circle, touch a red square.*
   30. *Put the green square next to the red circle.*
   31. *Touch the squares slowly and the circles quickly.*
   32. *Put the red circle between the yellow square and the green square.*
   33. *Touch all the circles, except the green one.*
   34. *Touch the red circle—no—the white square.*
   35. *Instead of the white square, touch the yellow circle.*
   36. *In addition to touching the yellow circle, touch the black circle.*

# 4

## Components of Auditory Comprehension: Analysis of Errors in a Revised Token Test

JAMES L. MACK AND FRANÇOIS BOLLER

The present study compares the performance of nonfluent and fluent aphasics with respect to two aspects of following spoken commands—selecting the designated stimuli and manipulating the stimuli in accordance with the syntactic relationships specified in the command—to determine whether or not these two groups showed qualitatively different patterns of impairment of comprehension. There has been considerable controversy in regard to the extent to which fluent and nonfluent aphasics can be differentiated on the basis of qualitative features of their performance on a comprehension task, although it is generally accepted that fluent aphasics are quantitatively more impaired than are nonfluents on such tasks. Goodglass, Gleason, and Hyde (1970) reported qualitatively different performances for fluent and nonfluent aphasics on comprehension of lexical elements (matching words to pictures) and more grammatically complex tasks (matching words to pictures denoting prepositional relationships). Such a finding is consistent with Luria's (1970) notion that comprehension of what he terms "logico-grammatical relationships" can be impaired independently of comprehension of lexical content. Subsequently, Heilman and Scholes (1976) found nonfluent (Wernicke's) aphasics to perform more poorly in matching the lexical elements of spoken sentences to pictures than were fluent (Broca's) and conduction aphasics, while there was no difference between the groups in making errors of syntactic comprehension. Recently Goodglass, Blumstein, Gleason, Green, Hyde, and Statlender (1977) compared the comprehension of these three aphasic subgroups on embedded sentences and on sentences with similar informational content which were disembedded and presented in an expanded version. Disembedding improved the performance of the nonfluent aphasics but had no effect on the performance of the other groups, leading the authors to interpret the comprehension deficit in nonfluent aphasia as based, at least in part, on a syntactic disorder. This conclusion has been supported by Schwartz, Saffran, and Marin (1978) who argued that nonfluent aphasics have a disorder of syntactic comprehension which is independent of the severity of their agrammatic output.

In contrast to the studies reviewed above, Parisi and Pizzamiglio (1970) asked subjects to match a spoken sentence to one of two pictures, using items which involved either phonemic, semantic, or syntactic discriminations, and found that while fluent and global aphasics were more impaired than nonfluents, when test items were scaled according to level of difficulty, the correlation between fluent and nonfluent aphasics was quite high ($r = .72$). Shewan and Canter (1971) used a similar procedure and varied syntactic difficulty (by using none, one, or two transformations), vocabulary level, and sentence length. Once again, fluent aphasics were more impaired than were nonfluents, but increased difficulty imposed by either syntactic complexity or vocabulary level had no qualitatively different effect on the aphasic subgroups.

While the conclusions of the studies just reviewed are clearly in opposition, the differences in procedures and materials are such that it is difficult to identify the basis of the discrepancies. It would be helpful if a familiar, clinically applicable test of comprehension could be used to evaluate the nature of the difference between the comprehension of fluent and nonfluent aphasics. In a recent review of auditory comprehension in aphasia, Boller, Kim, and Mack (1977) outlined the elements that should be included in an adequate test of auditory comprehension to evaluate the qualitative features of a subject's performance but commented that current tests of comprehension fail to include a number of necessary features. In the present study we determined to utilize an existing test, modified as necessary, to enable us to evaluate the subject's response to lexical and syntactic aspects of comprehension independently. Consistent with previous studies, we sought a test that did not require spoken responses, since nonfluent subjects were to be included. In addition, we wanted a test that would allow a wider scope for the spontaneous response of each subject so did not use a multiple choice or matching procedure, as has been used in most of the studies reviewed above. Therefore we selected a test in which the subject was asked to carry out a spoken command.

Perhaps the most widely used test involving spoken commands is the Token Test (De Renzi & Vignolo, 1962). It presents a series of spoken commands of increasing difficulty with a minimum of redundancy and has proved to be extremely sensitive to even mild aphasic deficits (cf. review in Boller *et al.*, 1977). The test as it is typically used, however, is not applicable to the present study, since each command, though including both lexical and—at the most difficult level—complex syntactic elements, is scored on an all or none basis. Furthermore, it has not been clear just what the Token Test measures and whether or not different aphasic subjects fail it for different reasons (Boller *et al.*, 1977).

Studies designed to identify the basis of aphasic deficits on the Token Test have not proved particularly fruitful. Several investigators have scaled the level of difficulty of Token Test items and found some parallels between the performance of aphasic adults and normal children (Whitaker & Noll, 1972; Poeck, Orgass, Kerschensteiner, & Hartje, 1974; Tallal, 1975). Since item difficulty levels for aphasics were not consistent across these studies, however, the hypotheses of Whitaker and Noll regarding the linguistic features of those items found to be most difficult in their study, must be regarded as quite tentative. Attempts have been made to explain Token Test performance as primarily dependent on attentional factors or sequencing span, which has been found to be related to Token Test performance in aphasics (Lesser, 1976; Tallal, 1975). Others, however, have minimized the contribution of attention or sequencing span to Token Test performance (Kreindler, Gheorghita, & Voinescu, 1971). Of even greater concern in regard to the utilization of the Token Test for the present study are the findings of Orgass and Poeck (1966) and Poeck, Hartje, Kerschensteiner, and Orgass (1973) who found that type of aphasia had no effect on overall Token Test scores. However, Kreindler *et al.* (1971) found Token Test deficits to be correlated with severity of receptive impairment though not with expressive impairment.

In view of the fact that Token Test studies have used items scored in the standard fashion, that is, right or wrong, it seems quite possible that any or all of the above reviewed studies may have obscured the relationships of comprehension ability, aphasia subtype, and sequencing span with item difficulty as measured by the lexical and syntactic aspects of the test items, if the hypothesis that lexical and syntactic aspects are relatively independent of one another is correct. Therefore, we designed the present study in order to evaluate the relative contribution of lexical and syntactic aspects of Token Test commands by modifying the scoring system of the test. Specifically we were interested in comparing the frequency of errors in touching the stimulus specified in a command (e.g., "Touch a *large red circle* and a *small white square*") with errors related to the more syntactic aspects of a command (e.g., "Touch a large red circle *after* you touch a small white square").

We made several modifications to the existing Token Test. First, we decided to emphasize the lexical and syntactic aspects by eliminating other sources of variance. Thus we used only one command, "touch," rather than including a variety of commands, such as "take," "put," etc., as are used in the standard version of the test. Furthermore, we decided to balance the stimulus elements more precisely than was done in the standard version in order to compare the relative difficulty imposed by each of the three attributes of the stimuli. This procedure has previously been used successfully by Kreindler *et al.* (1971). We also decided to add some syntactic aspects, such as "before" and "after," that have been considered to pose particular difficulty for some aphasics (Goodglass *et al.*, 1977; Luria, 1970). Finally, on the basis of a pilot study with normals, we eliminated a few commands from the standard version that had proved to be somewhat ambiguous and thus produced an inappropriately high error frequency among normals.

The present study was thus undertaken to test the following hypotheses:

1. There will be a greater frequency of errors in identifying the stimulus elements among fluent (Wernicke's) aphasics than among nonfluent (Broca's) aphasics.
2. There will be no difference in the frequency of errors between fluent and nonfluent aphasics in responding to the syntactic aspects of the commands, although both groups will make more syntactic errors than normal controls.

In order to ensure that our modifications in the Token Test had not changed the ability of the test to discriminate between aphasia per se and normal controls, we included the standard version of the Token Test and hypothesized that:

3. The Revised Token Test will discriminate between aphasics and normal controls as accurately as does the standard Token Test.

Since one previous study had balanced the stimulus attributes (Kreindler *et al.*, 1971) in the same manner as used in the present study, we sought to confirm their results by hypothesizing that:

4. The attribute of shape (square and circle) will produce more identification errors in the performance of aphasic subjects than will the attributes of size and color.

Finally, we performed an item analysis of the Revised Token Test to provide information regarding the respective difficulty level of the various syntactic elements of the commands in order to provide a basis for further modifications of the test in subsequent research.

## METHOD

*Subjects*

The normal control group consisted of 13 female hospital employees who voluntarily participated in the study. They ranged in age from 22 to 61 years, with a mean age of 38.69 ($SD = 13.19$). They all had had at least a high school education, with a mean of 13.15 years of school ($SD = 1.63$).

The aphasic group consisted of 15 aphasics (10 men and 5 women) being seen for either evaluation or treatment by the speech and audiology department of a county rehabilitation hospital or by a private hearing and speech center. Nearly all aphasics were outpatients, and all but one (who had a left temporal lobe tumor) had suffered aphasia as the result of a left hemisphere CVA. They were, as a group, significantly older than the control subjects, ranging in age from 53 to 72 years, with a mean age of 60.87 ($SD = 6.07$). Two of the aphasics had not completed high school, but their mean years of education was 12.79 ($SD = 3.49$), not significantly lower than that of the control group ($t = .34$). Nearly all aphasics were tested considerably past the onset of their symptoms, although two fluent aphasics were seen during the third month of their aphasia. The remainder had an onset of their aphasia from 4 to 88 months prior to testing, and all but one were receiving speech therapy at the time of testing.

The aphasics were divided into three subgroups on the basis of their evaluation by the speech program in which they were involved, supplemented by a brief aphasia screening test. Six were classified nonfluent with little or no clinical evidence of comprehension deficits;

three were nonfluent but also mildly impaired in their comprehension, and six were fluent with moderately to severely impaired comprehension.

*Materials*

The Token Test was presented in its commonly used format (Boller & Vignolo, 1966), except that squares were used instead of rectangles. The Revised Token Test, though based on the original, was modified to a considerable degree, particularly at the highest level, to facilitate the comparison of the influence of various aspects of the test on aphasic performance. In order to compare the difficulty of each stimulus attribute of the tokens themselves, only two examples of each identifying attribute were used. The stimuli were therefore reduced in number to eight tokens, with two colors (red and white) along with the two sizes (large and small) and shapes (square and circle) present in the original test. The lower levels of the revised test were essentially similar to those of the original, although individual commands were not identical.

The revised test was composed of seven levels, with the first five levels roughly corresponding to the first four levels in the Token Test. The subject was asked to "touch" a chip identified in Level I by only one stimulus attribute, for example, "red," in Level II by two attributes, for example, "large red," and in Level III by three attributes, for example, "large red square." In Level IV the subject was asked to touch two chips, each identified by two attributes, for example, a "large red" and a "small square" chip; while in Level V the subject was to touch two chips, each identified by all three stimulus attributes. Levels VI and VII of the revised test represent a considerable modification of the original test. All commands involving the comprehension of prepositions denoting spatial relationships among the stimuli were placed in Level VI and presented to subjects in three different ways. These results will be presented in a subsequent paper, however, and therefore will not be discussed further at present. Level VII represented commands of the type presented in Level V of the original Token Test except for commands dealing with locative prepositions. In order to further minimize the complexity of the commands so as to identify the basis for aphasic errors, the action required of the subject was reduced to a single act, that is, "touch," with the exception of two commands involving the use of "touch" in the overt instrumental sense, that is, "touch with," since this command has proved difficult for aphasics (Whitaker & Noll, 1972). The remainder of the commands in Level VII consisted of items using words denoting the order in which the command was to be carried out ("before," "after," "when"); the condition under which it was to be carried out ("if . . . then"); or other conjunctive words taken from the original test (e.g., "in addition to," "all except for," etc.). A number of items were presented in a transformed state, that is, passive or negative; and in some items the relationship of the order of words in the command and the order of action was reversed (e.g., "when I touch the . . . , you touch the . . ." versus "you touch the . . ., when I touch the . . .").

Each subject was given a nonverbal sequencing task. In this test the subject had to touch one at a time one or more of four 2.5 cm wooden cubes fixed in an horizontal array to a flat rectangular board 5 cm apart. On each trial the examiner touched a series of cubes (from one to seven) in a prescribed order, following which the subject was required to touch the cubes in the same sequence. If the subject failed an item, the demonstration was repeated once, but if the second trial was failed, the next item was administered. Four items were given at each level (i.e., number of cubes touched), from levels one to seven, and the test was discontinued when the subject failed both trials of all four items at a given level. Scores were assigned by giving two points for an item passed on the first trial and one point for a pass on the second trial, with these scores accumulated to a total weighted score which was used in the data analysis.

A brief aphasia screening test was administered to each subject in order to make sure normal controls were free from clinically evident aphasic deficits and to provide additional information to facilitate classification of aphasic subjects beyond that available from their speech pathology evaluations. Each subject was given a short series of simple commands and yes–no questions, a series of phrases and sentences of graduated length to be repeated, and a series of line drawings of common objects which he or she was to name or otherwise identify. From the results of these items and from observations of the subject's spontaneous speech, each subject was rated on a five point scale (no deficit to severely impaired) for each of four measures; comprehension, repetition, naming, and fluency.

Finally, each subject was given a verbal sequencing task. Instead of an array of four cubes, an array of four squares of the same dimensions, drawn on a single piece of 8.5 × 11 inch paper, each square having one of the numbers, 4, 3, 2, 1, ordered from left to right, was placed in front of the subject. The experimenter then spoke one or more of the numbers 1 through 4 aloud, corresponding exactly to the numerical equivalents of the cubes touched in the nonverbal sequencing task. The subject was then required to touch the numbered squares in an order corresponding to the numbers spoken by the experimenter. Thus the subject, in response to spoken numbers, made exactly the same movements as on the nonverbal task in order to complete a sequence correctly. This task was scored in the same manner as the nonverbal task.

*Procedure*

All subjects received the five tests in a fixed order, except that the two Token Tests were always given at the beginning and end of the testing session, with half of the subjects in each group receiving one first and the other last and half receiving the opposite order. The nonverbal sequencing test was given second, followed by the aphasia screening test and the verbal sequencing test. Most subjects were tested in a single session, lasting from 1 to 2 hours, but some aphasics could only be seen for 1 hour at a time and were therefore tested on two occasions, with the first two to four tests being given in the first session, depending on how quickly the subject proceeded.

## RESULTS

Scoring of the original Token Test followed the procedure of Spreen and Benton (1969), giving one point for each element of the command successfully followed. Scoring of the Revised Token Test was carried out in several ways. First, one point was awarded for the completion of each element of each command, the same procedure as was used for the Token Test. The results of this procedure were used for the comparison of the overall test scores of all subjects on the Token Test and the Revised Token Test presented in Table 4.1. On both the Token and Revised Token Tests, the six fluent aphasics fell to the bottom of the range of scores, while the control subjects were closely grouped near the top of the distribution. While the number of subjects was too small to permit any definitive conclusions regarding the utility of the two tests for differential diagnosis of aphasic subgroups, the revised test appeared to separate scores at the top end of the distribution to a greater degree than did the original Token Test. On the revised version the controls were distributed somewhat more widely ($p < .002$) and nonfluent aphasics with good comprehension showed less overlap with controls at the top of the aphasic range and less overlap with nonfluents with comprehension deficits at the bottom end of the nonfluent range than on the Token Test. It would appear reasonable to conclude that the Revised Token Test was not less diagnostically accurate than the original test and may be somewhat more useful in discriminating between aphasic subgroups

**TABLE 4.1**
*Distribution of Total Test Scores on Token Test and Revised Token Test for Aphasics and Normals*

| | Token Test | | | | | Revised Token Test | | | |
|---|---|---|---|---|---|---|---|---|---|
| Total score | N[a] | NF[b] | NF+[c] | F[d] | Total score | N | NF | NF+ | F |
| 320–325 | 13 | 4 | | | 360–365 | 10 | | | |
| 315–319 | | 1 | | | 355–359 | 3 | 1 | | |
| 310–314 | | 1 | 2 | | 350–354 | | 1 | | |
| 305–309 | | | | | 345–349 | | 3 | | |
| 300–304 | | | | | 340–344 | | | | |
| 295–399 | | | | | 335–339 | | | | |
| 290–294 | | | 1 | | 330–334 | | | | |
| 285–289 | | | | | 325–329 | | 1 | | |
| 280–284 | | | | | 320–324 | | | | |
| 275–279 | | | | | 315–319 | | | 1 | |
| 270–274 | | | | | 310–314 | | | | |
| 265–269 | | | | | 305–309 | | | 1 | |
| 260–264 | | | | 1 | 300–304 | | | | |
| 255–259 | | | | 1 | 295–299 | | | | |
| 250–254 | | | | | 290–294 | | | 1 | |
| 245–249 | | | | | 285–289 | | | | |
| 240–244 | | | | | 280–284 | | | | 1 |
| 235–239 | | | | 1 | 275–279 | | | | 1 |
| 230–234 | | | | | 270–274 | | | | |
| 225–229 | | | | | 265–269 | | | | |
| 220–224 | | | | | 260–264 | | | | |
| 215–219 | | | | | 255–259 | | | | |
| 210–214 | | | | | 250–254 | | | | |
| 205–209 | | | | | 245–249 | | | | |
| 200–204 | | | | | 240–244 | | | | 1 |
| 195–199 | | | | | 235–239 | | | | |
| 190–194 | | | | 1 | 230–234 | | | | |
| 185–189 | | | | | 225–229 | | | | 1 |
| 180–184 | | | | | 220–224 | | | | 1 |
| 175–179 | | | | | 215–219 | | | | |
| 170–174 | | | | 1 | 210–214 | | | | |
| 165–169 | | | | | 205–209 | | | | |
| 160–164 | | | | | 200–204 | | | | |
| 155–159 | | | | | 195–199 | | | | 1 |
| 150–154 | | | | 1 | 190–194 | | | | |

[a] N = 13 normal controls.
[b] NF = 6 nonfluent aphasics.
[c] NF+ = 3 nonfluent asphasics with comprehension deficits.
[d] F = 6 fluent asphasics.

as well as between aphasics with relatively good comprehension and normals.

Means and standard deviations of the controls and aphasics on the Token Tests and two measures of sequencing span are presented in Table 4.2. The aphasics were distinctly inferior to the controls on all measures. Aphasics, as a group, did much worse on both Token Tests and both sequencing tests than did normals. The Revised Token Test difference was of considerably greater statistical significance than that of the Token Test, perhaps reflecting the decreased overlap between groups seen on the revised test in Table 4.1.

The relationship of these scores is revealed in Table 4.3, which presents the intercorrelations between the same measures, along with age, a factor on which the two groups were clearly different. Age was not significantly correlated with any of the measures within either of the groups. Within the aphasic group the two Token Tests were highly correlated with one another, and both were highly correlated with performance on the verbal sequencing task, although correlation of either with the nonverbal sequencing task fell short of significance. Among the normal controls, performance on the two Token tests was not correlated, hardly unexpected in view of the restricted range of the control subjects on these two variables. Control performance on the Revised Token Test

**TABLE 4.2**
*Means and Standard Deviations on the Token Test, Revised Token Test, and Verbal and Nonverbal Sequencing Tests*

|  | Normals (N = 13) | Asphasics (N = 15) | t | df | Significance |
|---|---|---|---|---|---|
| Token Test |  |  |  |  |  |
| M | 324.15 | 274.20 | 3.06 | 26 | $p < .02$ |
| SD | .99 | 58.68 |  |  |  |
| Revised Token Test |  |  |  |  |  |
| M | 362.00 | 296.07 | 4.44 | 26 | $p < .002$ |
| SD | 2.89 | 53.31 |  |  |  |
| Verbal sequencing |  |  |  |  |  |
| M | 47.15 | 27.87 | 5.95 | 26 | $p < .002$ |
| SD | 6.53 | 9.96 |  |  |  |
| Nonverbal sequencing |  |  |  |  |  |
| M | 40.69 | 31.60 | 5.18 | 26 | $p < .002$ |
| SD | 5.42 | 3.83 |  |  |  |

**TABLE 4.3**
*Intercorrelations of Age, Token Test, Revised Token Test, and Verbal and Nonverbal Sequencing Test Performance for Normals (N = 13) and Aphasics (N = 15)*

|  |  | Token Test | Revised Token Test | Verbal sequencing | Nonverbal sequencing |
|---|---|---|---|---|---|
| Age | Normals | −.12 | −.13 | −.28 | −.43 |
|  | Aphasics | −.29 | −.19 | −.30 | −.31 |
| Token Test | Normals |  | .26 | .47 | .09 |
|  | Aphasics |  | .95*** | .86*** | .50 |
| Revised Token Test | Normals |  |  | .66* | .38 |
|  | Aphasics |  |  | .86*** | .37 |
| Verbal sequencing | Normals |  |  |  | .71** |
|  | Aphasics |  |  |  | .49 |

*$p < .05$.
**$p < .01$.
***$p < .001$.

was mildly correlated with verbal sequencing, while the Token Test correlation with verbal sequencing fell just short of significance. Finally, performance on the two sequencing tasks was correlated among controls but fell short of significance among the aphasics.

For the major analysis of the present study, Revised Token Test performance was scored separately for stimulus errors and syntactic errors. A stimulus error consisted of touching a stimulus other than the one specified in the command, while a syntactic error consisted of failing that part of the command not involving the identification of the stimulus by its attributes but concerned with those features described above related to the order in which the stimuli were touched, etc. Syntactic errors could occur only on Levels VI (not here reported) and VII, while stimulus errors could occur at any level.

In many instances on Level VII judgments could be made about syntactic and stimulus errors independently, while in some cases, particularly with grossly deviant responses, judgments could not be made about one or another feature of the subject's response. Each test item was thus scored in terms that applied to that item alone.

Stimulus identification and syntactic errors made by all subjects are presented in Table 4.4. It should be noted that a few stimulus errors and a fair number of syntactic errors were observed among the control subjects. While several of the nonfluent aphasics with good comprehension made no stimulus errors, all made syntactic errors, and only two made so

**TABLE 4.4**
*Revised Token Test: Types of Errors Made by Normals and Aphasics*

|  | Subject | Revised Token Test Total | Stimulus errors | Syntactic errors |
|---|---|---|---|---|
| Normals | 1 | 365 | 0 | 0 |
|  | 2 | 365 | 0 | 0 |
|  | 3 | 365 | 0 | 0 |
|  | 4 | 365 | 0 | 0 |
|  | 5 | 364 | 0 | 1 |
|  | 6 | 364 | 0 | 1 |
|  | 7 | 363 | 0 | 2 |
|  | 8 | 360 | 0 | 1 |
|  | 9 | 360 | 1 | 5 |
|  | 10 | 360 | 4 | 0 |
|  | 11 | 359 | 0 | 2 |
|  | 12 | 359 | 1 | 5 |
|  | 13 | 357 | 0 | 4 |
| Nonfluents | 1 | 356 | 1 | 5 |
|  | 2 | 352 | 8 | 3 |
|  | 3 | 349 | 0 | 12 |
|  | 4 | 348 | 0 | 13 |
|  | 5 | 345 | 4 | 7 |
|  | 6 | 328 | 12 | 10 |
| Nonfluents with comprehension deficits | 7 | 316 | 23 | 10 |
|  | 8 | 305 | 19 | 14 |
|  | 9 | 294 | 17 | 16 |
| Fluents | 10 | 284 | 34 | 15 |
|  | 11 | 278 | 42 | 12 |
|  | 12 | 241 | 40 | 18 |
|  | 13 | 226 | 52 | 23 |
|  | 14 | 221 | 64 | 19 |
|  | 15 | 198 | 64 | 31 |

few syntactic errors as to fall within the upper limits of the control distribution. In contrast, the nonfluents with comprehension deficits and the fluents made a considerable number of stimulus errors as well as syntactic errors. The relative frequencies of each type of error on Level VII within the four groups are best seen in Figure 4.1. While the mean number of syntactic errors shows a steady increase across the four groups, with clear overlap between the aphasic subgroups, the mean number of stimulus errors shows a distinct increase in the fluent aphasics, with maximum overlap between the controls and the nonfluents with good comprehension.

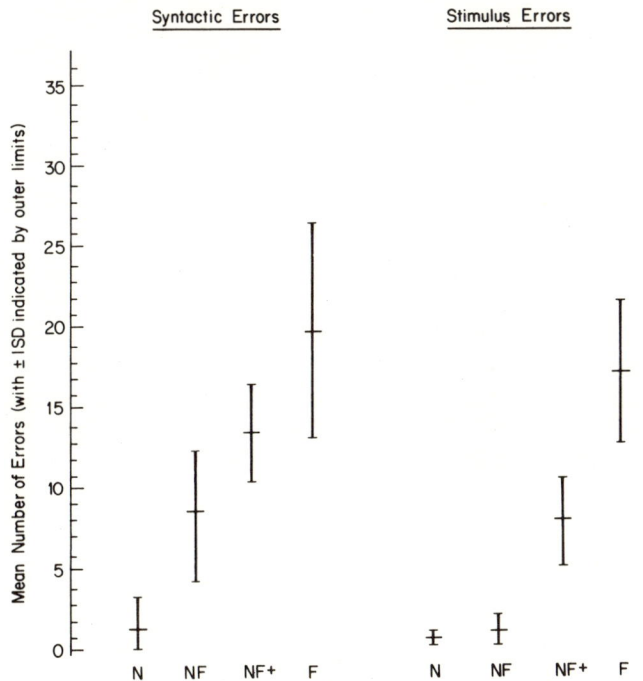

**FIGURE 4.1.** *Revised Token Test: Level VII. Means and standard deviations of three aphasic groups for syntactic and stimulus errors. N = 13 normal controls, NF = 6 nonfluent aphasics, NF+ = 3 nonfluent aphasics with comprehension deficits, and F = 6 fluent aphasics.*

The significance of the difference in the frequency of stimulus and syntactic errors between the groups on Level VII of the Revised Token Test was calculated by means of the Mann-Whitney $U$ test. The fluent aphasics made significantly more stimulus identification errors than did controls ($p < .002$), nonfluent aphasics with good comprehension ($p < .002$), or nonfluents with comprehension deficits ($p = .024$). The nonfluents with poor comprehension also made significantly more errors than did controls ($p < .02$) or nonfluents with good comprehension ($p = .024$). The nonfluents with good comprehension and the controls, while making significantly less errors than the other aphasic groups, were not significantly different from one another with respect to accuracy of stimulus identification. Results relating to the frequency of syntactic errors followed a different pattern. The fluent aphasics made significantly more syntactic errors than did the control subjects ($p < .002$) or the nonfluent aphasics with good comprehension ($p = .006$). The nonfluents with poor comprehension made more errors than controls ($p < .02$) but were not significantly different from either of the other aphasic groups. The nonfluent aphasics with good comprehension, though performing at a more accurate level than the fluent aphasics, made significantly more syntactic errors than did the control subjects ($p < .002$).

The frequencies of stimulus and syntactic errors for individual aphasics were clearly related. The correlation between the total number of syntactic and stimulus errors for each aphasic on the 27 items of Level VII where both syntactic and stimulus errors could occur was .81. On the other hand, the correlation between the number of subjects making syntactic errors and the number making stimulus errors on each item was insignificant ($r = .16$). That is, although the number of stimulus errors made by a given subject was highly related to the number of syntactic errors made by that subject, the number of subjects failing the syntactic aspect of a given item was not related to the number of subjects failing the stimulus aspect of that item. When the 27 items on which both syntactic and stimulus errors could be made were scaled in order of difficulty for the two types of errors, the correlation between orders of difficulty was insignificant ($r = .18$). It should be noted that the order of difficulty for either syntactic or stimulus errors was not significantly correlated with the order of administration of the items on Level VII.

Stimulus errors of aphasic subjects on each level of the Revised Token Test are presented in Table 4.5. Note that in the comparisons of syntactic and stimulus error frequencies made above, a stimulus error was scored only once for a single item on Level VII, to make the number comparable to the syntactic errors which could only be scored once per item. In the following analysis, however, since the contribution of each attribute is to be considered, each stimulus to be identified is scored for each attribute designated in the command. Thus a stimulus designated by three attributes could produce as many as three stimulus errors. The column totals of Table 4.5 indicate the total number of stimulus errors made on each level of the Revised Token Test. When the actual frequency of stimulus errors at each level was compared to the expected frequency of errors (based on the number of possible errors, which were different for each level), the difference in error frequencies across levels was highly significant by $\chi^2$ test ($p < .001$). The first three levels showed fewer errors than would be expected, while the last five were not significantly different from their expected level. Exactly the same pattern of results was obtained if only one stimulus error was counted for each token to be touched. Thus the significant increase in error frequency occurred in the transition from Level III to Level IV with the introduction of a second stimulus to be touched. In Level III the subject is asked

**TABLE 4.5**
*Stimulus Errors as a Function of Test Level for Asphasics*

| Error type | | I | II | III | IV | V | VIb | VIc | VII | Total | Grand total |
|---|---|---|---|---|---|---|---|---|---|---|---|
| Large to small | NF[a] | | | | | | 1 | 1 | 1 | 3 | |
| | NF+[b] | | | | | 2 | | 1 | 2 | 5 | 46 |
| | F[c] | | 1 | 2 | 2 | 5 | 10 | 18 | 38 | | |
| Small to large | NF | | | | | | | 1 | 1 | 2 | |
| | NF+ | | | | 1 | 2 | 3 | | 4 | 10 | 50 |
| | F | | | | 3 | 2 | 4 | 15 | 14 | 38 | |
| Red to white | NF | | | | | | | | | 0 | |
| | NF+ | | | | | 2 | | 1 | 3 | 6 | 56 |
| | F | | | 2 | 4 | 7 | 7 | 13 | 17 | 50 | |
| White to red | NF | | | | | | | 1 | | 1 | |
| | NF+ | | | | | | 2 | 5 | 2 | 9 | 63 |
| | F | | 1 | 1 | 1 | 4 | 7 | 15 | 24 | 53 | |
| Square to circle | NF | | | | | 2 | 2 | 3 | 4 | 11 | |
| | NF+ | | | | | 3 | 4 | 5 | 10 | 22 | 106 |
| | F | | | 3 | | 3 | 13 | 9 | 21 | 24 | 73 | |
| Circle to square | NF | | | | 1 | 2 | 2 | 2 | 1 | 8 | |
| | NF+ | 1 | | 1 | 1 | | | 3 | 1 | 7 | 59 |
| | F | 1 | | | 4 | 3 | 8 | 12 | 16 | 44 | |
| Totals by group | NF | | | | 1 | 4 | 5 | 8 | 7 | 25 | |
| | NF+ | 1 | | 1 | 2 | 9 | 9 | 15 | 22 | 59 | |
| | F | 1 | 4 | 4 | 17 | 31 | 40 | 86 | 113 | 296 | |
| Grand total | | 2 | 4 | 5 | 20 | 44 | 54 | 109 | 142 | 380 | |

[a]NF = Nonfluents ($N = 6$).
[b]NF+ = Nonfluents with comprehension deficit ($N = 3$).
[c]F = Fluents ($N = 6$).

to touch, for example, "a large white circle," while in Level IV the subject must touch, for example, "a large circle and a white square." Apparent increases in error frequencies beyond Level IV are simply due to the increased number of possible errors.

The next feature of Table 4.5, shown in the row totals, relates to the effect of the stimulus attributes. A $\chi^2$ test of the grand totals in the right hand column indicated that shape produced far more errors than other stimulus attributes ($p < .001$). In particular, "square" was misidentified significantly more often than all other stimulus attributes, which were not significantly different from one another in terms of frequency of misidentification. The numbers of each attribute within the commands were equal, so that this difference does not reflect differing frequencies of occurrence of each attribute.

The role of the various syntactic features of the Revised Token Test was evaluated in an item analysis in which the proportion of control and aphasic subjects passing each item of Level VII (without regard for stimulus errors) were compared in order to determine the most discriminating items. These results, of course, would require cross validation in a separate group of subjects, before they could be applied to clinical use. It should be noted that this type of item analysis, in which the most discriminating items are identified, is different from that carried out by other investigators (e.g., Whitaker & Noll, 1972; Poeck, Orgass, Kerschensteiner, & Hartje, 1974), who simply examined the frequency of aphasics who failed each item on the highest level of the Token Test.

All discrimination indices were represented by a proportion, reflecting the number of control subjects who passed the item plus the number of aphasics who failed the item, divided by the total number of subjects ($N = 28$). All four commands asking the subject to touch a stimulus "when" the experimenter touched another stimulus were highly discriminating. The two commands with the "when" clause in the initial position in the command appeared to be more difficult than the two commands with the "when" clause in the final position (.79 and .89 versus .68 and .79, respectively). Furthermore, if the "when" clause was transformed to the passive (e.g., "When the large red square has been touched by me, you touch the..."), the commands appeared to be more discriminating than their active counterparts (.89 and .79 versus .79 and .68, respectively). "Before" clauses, which always appeared in the initial position of a command, thus requiring the subject to reverse the order in which the command was to be carried out, seemed more difficult than "after" clauses, which also were presented in the initial position and thus entailed no reversal of the action from the order of the command (.75, .68, and .86 versus .68, .57, and .79, respectively). The discrimination level of both "before" and "after" clauses was apparently enhanced by using an embedded construction (e.g., "Before you touch the chip I touch, touch the..."), which yielded the highest discrimination indices of these six commands (.79 and .86). Eight items using a conditional ("If...") command showed a wide range of discrimination indices (from .54 to .79), although the two most discriminating commands both involved an embedded construction (.75 and .79). Two commands using the verb "touch" in the overt instrumental sense ("touch with") were also highly discriminating (.75 and .79). While very simple embedded clauses ("Touch the chip I touch.") proved to be of little difficulty for the aphasics, double embedded commands ("Touch the chip I touch that is white.") were somewhat more discriminating (.64), although their discriminatory effectiveness suffered because the controls occasionally made errors, probably due to the apparent ambiguity of the item. Finally a command asking the subject to touch one chip "in addition to" another (.75) and two commands asking the subject to touch "all the . . . except for the . . ." (.71 and .82) were also effective in discriminating between aphasics and controls.

Nondiscriminating items included "Touch the . . ., No!—touch the . . ." (.54), "Touch the . . . but not the . . . " (.54), "Instead of the . . ., touch the . . ." (.50), and the simple embedded sentences described above (.54 and .50). All of these were passed by nearly all aphasics, perhaps by ignoring the linguistic complexity of the items and simply touching the last named token or imitating the examiner's action.

Analyzing the effect of the syntactic aspects of the commands by means of a discrimination index produced minimal changes from what would have resulted using the previously reported type of item analysis, that is, simply ranking the items in the order of difficulty for aphasic subjects. Three commands, a "when" clause, an item using touch in the overt instrumental sense, and the two commands using a double embedded sentence would have been considered more powerful using the simpler method of analysis, but their discrimination indices were reduced by a relatively high proportion of errors among the control subjects, although no item was failed by more than 5 of the 13 controls.

## DISCUSSION

The results of the present study clearly confirm the first hypothesis since fluent aphasics made considerably more errors in identifying the stimulus elements than did the nonfluent aphasics with good comprehension or the normal control subjects. Both controls and nonfluents with good comprehension made some stimulus errors and were not significantly different from one another, but the mean total error scores in Figure 4.1 reveal a striking disparity between the results of the fluent aphasics and the other aphasic subjects. The nonfluent aphasics with poor comprehension, while significantly superior to the fluents, also made significantly more stimulus errors than either the controls or the remaining nonfluents. These results are quite consistent with those of

Heilman and Scholes (1976). In view of the fact that most tests of comprehension rely primarily on comprehension of lexical items, as Heilman and Scholes point out, it is not surprising that fluent aphasics do so poorly and nonfluents so well on these tests. The comprehension problem of the nonfluents with poor comprehension seems to be, at least in part, similar to that of the fluent aphasics, in the sense that both groups are distinguished from normals and nonfluent aphasics with good comprehension by the number of stimulus errors they make.

The second hypothesis, that there would be no difference in the frequency of syntactic errors between the fluent and nonfluent aphasics, was only partly supported. While stimulus errors clearly divided the aphasics into three distinct groups and failed to distinguish between normal controls and nonfluents with good comprehension, syntactic errors distinguished all aphasic groups from normals but also partially separated the three aphasic subgroups in the present study. Fluent aphasics did make significantly more syntactic errors than did the nonfluents with good comprehension, who, in turn, made more errors than normals. The nonfluents with poor comprehension fell between the performance levels of the other aphasic groups and were significantly different from neither.

In contrast to the present results, Heilman and Scholes found no difference between subtypes of aphasics on the syntactic aspects of a different type of sentence-comprehension task. Their syntactic task required the subject to distinguish between the direct and indirect objects in a spoken sentence in order to match the sentence to a picture which showed the correct relationship and was contrasted with another picture which had the objects reversed. Two remaining pictures showed incorrect objects in direct and indirect relationships. Selecting either of the two latter pictures was scored as a lexical (stimulus identification) error, while selecting the initial contrast was scored as a syntactic error. Thus the task was different from the present design in three ways: The subject had to match a spoken sentence to a picture in a multiple-choice format; results were scored in such a fashion that making one type of error precluded making the other type; and finally, only one type of syntactic manipulation was used, the relationship conveyed by the direct or indirect object, while the present study included a much larger number of syntactic components, which, among themselves, varied considerably in the extent to which they proved to be difficult for the aphasics. The differences between the present study and that of Heilman and Scholes (1976) are so great, that the results can hardly be regarded as contradictory.

The present results clearly support the importance of examining the semantic or lexical and syntactic aspects of aphasic comprehension independently. The particular aspect to be emphasized in a specific investigation would depend on the goal of the study. If one wishes to distinguish between aphasics and normals, elements with a high degree of syntactic complexity, much like those of the original Token Test, should function as the most significant discriminators. On the other hand, if one wishes to differentiate subgroups of aphasics, a task for which the original Token Test has been considered of little utility (e.g., Orgass & Poeck, 1966), items with a high degree of lexical difficulty and minimal syntactic complexity would probably yield the most accurate results. In this respect, it should be noted that most aphasia batteries include comprehension items that are best used for the latter type of discrimination, and most aphasia batteries have been designed to provide a detailed diagnosis of the type of aphasia rather than to distinguish aphasics from normals. Nevertheless, modification of the Token Test by allowing the independent evaluation of stimulus or lexical and syntactic errors seems to hold the promise of performing both discrimination tasks with the same instrument. From a theoretical point of view, the present study supports the notion that different aphasic groups have qualitatively different patterns of comprehension impairment.

The third hypothesis was strongly confirmed. The Revised Token Test was at least as effective as the Token Test, scored according to the technique of Spreen and Benton (1969), in discriminating aphasics from normal controls, and total scores for the two tests were very highly correlated. There did appear to be a suggestion of differences in the dispersion of normal and aphasic scores on the two tests, however. Although both tests produced few errors among the control subjects, their performance on the revised test was more varied than on the original test. More important, there appeared to be less overlap between aphasic subtypes and, at the same time, less overlap between the least impaired aphasics and the controls on the revised test in comparison with the original version. While these differences were based on too small a sample size to be immediately generalizable for clinical purposes, they certainly indicate that the modifications have not had the effect of diminishing the clinical utility of the test but instead may have enhanced it. Why this might be so is suggested in the results concerning the relationship between aspects of comprehension and aphasic subtype. The revised test contained a larger proportion of items based on syntactic difficulty than did the original. The Token Test consists of 62 items, 40 (the first four levels) of which have little syntactic complexity. In contrast the Revised

Token Test included only 20 of 77 items at such a reduced level of syntactic complexity. Thus, the larger number of syntactically difficult items may have caused the increased effectiveness of the revised test in separating aphasics from normals, since syntactic errors appear to be the most effective means of performing this discrimination.

More surprising is the observation that the Revised Token Test also seemed to separate the aphasic subgroups from one another more accurately than the original test, in spite of the fact that the revised test contained a proportionally smaller total of possible stimulus errors than the original; and stimulus errors were found to be the most effective means of discriminating aphasic subtypes. There was no indication that this apparently enhanced separation of aphasic subtypes could have been due to some subtle interaction of syntactic and stimulus errors. As the syntactic demands of the task increased (i.e., in Levels VI and VII), stimulus errors did not become more frequent. Apparently the incidence of stimulus errors is so small among the nonfluent aphasics with good comprehension, that the proportion of stimulus errors in the revised test, though smaller than in the original, is still sufficient to separate the aphasic subgroups in terms of total test scores.

Analysis of the types of stimulus errors made by the aphasics indicated that the frequency of errors for the three stimulus attributes was not equal. Errors were made far more frequently in regard to the attribute of shape than in regard to size or color, thus confirming the fourth hypothesis and supporting the earlier findings of Kreindler *et al.* (1971), who also demonstrated that the increase in errors for the attribute of shape was not due to serial position in the command. In particular, the errors due to shape in the present study were due to erroneous responses to "square," while "circle" produced no more errors than other stimulus attributes. Why "square" should be more difficult than the other five attributes is not clear. Whitaker and Whitaker (this volume) have noted that both "circle" and "square" have lower frequencies in English usage than the other attributes used in the present test. The frequency of "circle," however, is lower than that of "square" so that frequency is not a sufficient explanation of the difficulty imposed by "square."

Perhaps the most difficult question that must be dealt with concerns the relationship of primary memory and auditory comprehension. The present study confirms previous work reporting a significant relationship between tests of sequencing span and Token Test performance. Both the original and revised tests were highly correlated with a test of verbal sequencing span among the aphasics ($r = .86$ for both Token Tests) but not significantly correlated with a test of nonverbal sequencing span ($r = .50$ for the original and .38 for the revised). Lesser (1976) found Token Test performance to be correlated with performance on a verbal sequencing task as well as, though to a smaller degree, on a less verbal sequencing task, but she did not report the degree of correlation. She argued that since aphasics made errors in earlier levels of the Token Test, where the amount of information fell within their verbal sequencing span, all of their errors could not be attributed to primary memory impairment, but that, since the most syntactically demanding part of the test, Level V, presented information that exceeded the aphasics' sequencing span, the Token Test could not be used to draw conclusions regarding the influence of syntactic factors on aphasic performance. The present results confirm Lesser's distinction between aphasic performance on a verbal sequencing task, on which they were most impaired, and a relatively nonverbal task, on which they were impaired to a smaller extent, thus arguing against the position supported by the work of Kimura and Archibald (1974) that left hemisphere damaged aphasics may be impaired on all motor sequencing tasks to a similar degree.

On the other hand, the present results do not entirely agree with Lesser's notion that the relationship between verbal sequencing span and Token Test performance preclude the analysis of syntactic contributions to the Token Test performance of aphasics. In the present study, the major effect of span difficulties was seen in the transition from Level III, in which the subject was asked to touch a single token identified by three attributes, to Level IV of the Revised Token Test, in which the subject was asked to touch two tokens, each identified by two stimulus attributes. Adding a third attribute to designate each of two tokens (as in Level V of the revised test) did not significantly increase the frequency of stimulus errors. In other words, either adding a third attribute to designate the stimuli to be touched did not increase the information load or the frequency of stimulus errors is not necessarily affected by increases in information load, despite the high correlation between verbal sequencing span and Revised Token Test performance among the aphasics. It seems possible that even when the sequencing span of an aphasic subject is taxed by the presentation of information presumably exceeding his span, the patient may nevertheless follow a command accurately enough to allow the evaluation of specific aspects of his performance.

When only items at the most difficult level in terms of information load, that is, Level VII, were considered, the total number of stimulus errors made by an aphasic was closely related to the total number of syntactic errors made by the subject, yet the stimulus or syntactic difficulty of each item, judged in terms of the frequency with which subjects failed either the stimulus or syntactic aspects of the command, were not correlated. Thus some items presumably reflected syntactic difficulty, others, semantic difficulty (i.e., errors of stimulus identification). Furthermore, although overall Revised Token Test performance among the aphasics was highly correlated with verbal sequencing span and errors of both types occurred primarily at the highest test levels (V through VII), the three subgroups of aphasics produced significantly different numbers of stimulus errors compared to one another, while they were far less different in terms of the number of syntactic errors they produced, indicating qualitatively different patterns of impairment, in spite of the fact that on Levels V through VII their span of attention was presumably being overly taxed. Thus, it seems reasonable to conclude that the syntactic contribution of test items can be evaluated, even though verbal sequencing span ability is undoubtedly an important contributor to Revised Token Test performance among the aphasics.

The question of the meaning of the very high correlation ($r = .86$) between verbal sequencing span and Revised Token Test performance remains to be explored. It may well be that primary memory span for verbal material and auditory comprehension are inextricably interrelated. The next logical extention of the present results lies in comparing the performance of patients with left and right unilateral hemisphere damage to determine to what extent the "syntactic" difficulties of the aphasics may be due to brain damage per se rather than to damage specifically localized within the left hemisphere. It may well be that right hemisphere patients will also have impairments related to this aspect of Revised Token Test performance. We are currently collecting data on comparable groups of left and right hemisphere lesioned subjects to answer this question.

Item analysis of Revised Token Test items revealed that not all items appeared to effectively discriminate between aphasics and normal controls. Several items taken from the original Token Test proved to be insufficiently difficult, even for severely impaired fluent aphasics, and it was suggested that these items were probably being solved by simply ignoring the syntactic complexity of the command. In contrast, a number of items seem to be effective discriminators between aphasics and controls, including items using clauses beginning with "when," "before," "after," "if," "all . . . except for"; the conjunction "in addition to"; and "with" in the overt instrumental sense. In addition to the effect of specific clauses, several manipulations seemed to pose difficulties for the aphasics. In particular, syntactic errors seemed to be increased by the use of embedding (consistent with the findings of Goodglass *et al.*, 1977) and by presenting clauses in which the order of the command was the reverse of the sequence in which the action had to be carried out. None of the tentative findings related to the syntactic difficulties imposed by particular types of constructions and words can as yet be regarded as conclusive findings, although several of the results were consistent with the findings of previous investigators. We are now engaged in a study of the influence of various syntactic modifications of the items found to be effective discriminators in the present study; we are systematically varying such factors as the relationship of the order in which the stimuli are designated in the command with the order in which the stimuli are touched in carrying out the action, the number of attributes used to designate the stimulus to be touched, and the effect of the intrusion of an intervening action by the experimenter in following a command.

It is our hope that the next study will provide a basis for constructing a clinically useful instrument that will enable us to distinguish between aphasics and normals and between various aphasic subtypes in terms of stimulus and syntactic errors scored independently. In addition, the data we collect should provide some understanding of the type of syntactic modifications that pose particular difficulty for aphasics and for patients with right hemisphere lesions and thus yield further insights into the relationship between specific aspects of auditory comprehension and brain function.

## ACKNOWLEDGMENTS

We wish to thank Nancy Spence of the Cleveland Hearing and Speech Center and Paul Langman and the remainder of the staff of the Speech and Audiology Department of Highland View Hospital for their help in providing us with the patients who are the subjects of this study. In addition we wish to acknowledge the help of Kay Gorman, Andrea Mack, and Jean Moise, who spent considerable time in testing the subjects.

## APPENDIX

Revised Token Test Items[a]

I.    1. *Touch a small one.*
      2. *Touch a red one.*

[a]The following abbreviations are used in designating the stimuli on the list of test items:

    S-small    R-red    Cir-circle
    L-large    W-white    Sq-square

The stimuli were always arranged in two horizontal rows, so that subject, when facing the examiner across a table, saw on the table between them the following arrangement of tokens, from subject's left to right:

    Examiner
    LRSq, SRCir, SRSq, LWCir
    SWCir, LWSq, LRCir, SWSq
    Subject

|      |    |                                                                                              |
|------|----|----------------------------------------------------------------------------------------------|
|      | 3. | *Touch a square.*                                                                            |
|      | 4. | *Touch a white one.*                                                                         |
|      | 5. | *Touch a circle.*                                                                            |
|      | 6. | *Touch a large one.*                                                                         |
| II.  | 1. | *Touch a small square.*                                                                      |
|      | 2. | *Touch a large white one.*                                                                   |
|      | 3. | *Touch a red circle.*                                                                        |
| III. | 1. | *Touch a small white circle.*                                                                |
|      | 2. | *Touch a large red square.*                                                                  |
|      | 3. | *Touch a large white square.*                                                                |
|      | 4. | *Touch a small red circle.*                                                                  |
| IV.  | 1. | *Touch a white circle and a large red one.*                                                  |
|      | 2. | *Touch a red square and a small circle.*                                                     |
|      | 3. | *Touch a small white one and a large square.*                                                |
| V.   | 1. | *Touch a large white square and a small red square.*                                         |
|      | 2. | *Touch a small white circle and a large red square.*                                         |
|      | 3. | *Touch a small red circle and a small white square.*                                         |
|      | 4. | *Touch a large white circle and a large red circle.*                                         |
| VI. A | 1. | *Touch the chip next to the small white circle.*                                            |
|       | 2. | *Touch the chip between the large red square and the small red square.*                     |
|       | 3. | *Touch the chip closest to the large white circle.*                                         |
|       | 4. | *Touch the chip below the small red circle.*                                                |
|       | 5. | *Touch the chip beside the small white square.*                                             |
|       | 6. | *Touch the chip farthest from the large white square.*                                      |
|       | 7. | *Touch the chip above the large red circle.*                                                |
|       | 8. | *Touch the chip that is closer to the large red square than the small white circle is.*     |
| VI. B | 1. | *Put the blue chip next to the small white circle.*                                         |
|       | 2. | *Put the blue chip between the large white square and the small red square.*                |
|       | 3. | *Put the blue chip closest to the large white circle.*                                      |
|       | 4. | *Put the blue chip below the small red circle.*                                             |
|       | 5. | *Put the blue chip beside the small white square.*                                          |
|       | 6. | *Put the blue chip farthest from the large white square.*                                   |
|       | 7. | *Put the blue chip above the large red circle.*                                             |
|       | 8. | *Put the blue chip closer to the large red square than the small white circle is.*          |
| VI. C | 1. | *Put the large red circle next to the small white circle.*                                  |
|       | 2. | *Put the large white circle between the large white square and the small red square.*       |
|       | 3. | *Put the large red square closest to the large white circle.*                               |
|       | 4. | *Put the small white square below the small red circle.*                                    |
|       | 5. | *Put the small red square beside the small white square.*                                   |
|       | 6. | *Put the small red circle farthest from the large white square.*                            |
|       | 7. | *Put the small white circle above the large red circle.*                                    |
|       | 8. | *Put the large white square closer to the large red square than the small white circle is.* |
| VII.  | 1. | *Touch the chip that I touch* (LRCir).                                                      |
|       | 2. | *When I touch the large red square, you touch the small white square.* (SRCir, pause, LW square, paus, **LR Sq,** pause—then continue if no response, SWCir) |
|       | 3. | *Instead of the small white square, touch the large white circle.*                          |
|       | 4. | *Touch the large white square but not the large red circle.*                                |

5. Touch all the red ones, beginning with the small circle.
6. If you are a woman, touch the large white circle.
7. If you are not a woman, touch the large red square.
8. Before touching the large white square, touch the small white circle.
9. Touch the large white circle, when I touch the small red circle. (**SRCir,** pause—then continue if no response, LR Sq, pause, SWCir)
10. Touch all the small ones, except for the red square.
11. Touch the small white circle. No! Touch the large white square.
12. The chip that I touch, you touch. (SW Sq)
13. In addition to the large white circle, touch the small red circle.
14. Touch the chip that I touch that is white, (SR Sq, pause, **SWCir,** pause, LRCir).
15. If you are not an American, touch the chip that I touch. (SRCir)
16. If you are an American, touch the chip that I touch. (SW Sq)
17. Beginning with the large red one, touch all the circles.
18. When the small red square has been touched by me, you touch the small white circle. (SW Sq, pause, **SR Sq,** pause—then continue if no response, LRCir)
19. After you touch the small red circle, touch the chip that I touch. (LR Sq)
20. Touch either the large red circle or the small red square.
21. After touching the large red circle, touch the small white square.
22. Touch the chip that I touch that is large. (SRCir, pause, **LR Sq,** pause, SWCir)
23. After the large white circle has been touched by me, you touch the large red square.
24. If the chip that I touch is red (LW Sq) touch the small white square.
25. If the chip that I touch is small (SWCir) touch the large red circle.
26. Except for the large white one, touch all the squares.
27. Before the small red circle has been touched by me, you touch the large white circle.
28. Touch the large white square, when the large red circle has been touched by me. (LR Sq, pause, **LRCir,** pause—then continue if no response, SWCir)
29. Before you touch the small red square, touch the chip that I touch. (LRCir)
30. Touch the large white square, if the chip that I touch is large. (SR Sq)
31. Touch the small red square, if the chip that I touch is a circle. (SWCir)
32. Touch the small red circle with the large red square.
33. With the small white circle, touch the small red square.

# 5

## Turning Tokens into Things: Linguistic and Mnestic Aspects of the Initial Sections of the Token Test

RUTH LESSER

Studies of the Token Test with adults fall, in general, into two categories. First, there are those concerned with its validation and refinement as a clinical instrument which distinguishes aphasics from nonaphasics and establishes the degree of deficit in comprehension. Second, there are those that search for the components in the test (in its various parts and versions) which contribute to its diagnostic efficiency. Such studies provide an avenue for the better understanding of the pathology of higher cortical functions. They use the test, not as a device for the assessment of aphasic individuals, but as a means of investigating aphasia as such. The present study falls into this category.

The test appears to include components which make it sensitive to all types of aphasia, regardless of locus of lesion (Orgass & Poeck, 1966; Poeck, Kerschensteiner, & Hartje, 1972; Cohen, Kelter, Engel, List, & Strohner, 1976), and even to left-hemisphere damage without overt aphasia (Boller, 1968; Boller & Vignolo, 1966). Leischner (1974) lists, among the components which make the Token Test so susceptible, the artificiality of the test situation, the test's vulnerability to failures of attention and concentration, to fatigue and to optic-gnostic disturbances, and the difficulty of differentiating a rapid series of similar tasks. The test's authors (De Renzi & Vignolo, 1962) suggested other components: the lack of redundancy of the message transmitted; and a possible specific difficulty with geometric shape names due to their late age of acquisition and the ambiguity of their grammatical status as nouns or adjectives. Kreindler, Gheorghita, and Voinescu (1971) found evidence that the abstract nature of the tokens contributed to the difficulty of the Token Test. Another component that has been proposed is the test's dependency on visuo-spatial skills (Swisher & Sarno, 1969). Other contributing factors include a subject's cognitive ability to analyze a whole into its elements (Cohen, Kelter, & Schäfer, 1977), as well as his reliance on verbal and nonverbal memory, particularly for sequences (Lesser, 1976; Scolaro & Flowers, 1977).

A further stimulus to investigation has been the observation that one section of the test (Part V, which includes grammatical features such as predication, subordination, and locative adverbial phrases) seems to be as good a discriminator of aphasia as is the whole test (Boller & Vignolo, 1966; Hartje, Kerschensteiner, Poeck, & Orgass, 1973; Sipos, & Tägert, 1972). Explanations have been offered in terms of a distinctively aphasic difficulty with decoding particles and interstitial words (Zaidel, 1977) and in terms of the variability of the implicit case relations of the verbs used (Poeck, Orgass, Kerschensteiner, & Hartje, 1974; Whitaker & Noll, 1972). Lesser (1976) found a significant correlation of Part V with a measure of the organization of nonverbal gestural sequences. There have been suggestions that the left hemisphere is particularly associated with the organization of motor sequences, and with the control of transitions from one posture to another (Kimura, 1973, 1977). Lesser therefore argued against the simple interpretation of aphasic errors in Part V in linguistic terms, as if it were a pure test of verbal comprehension. These errors appear, rather, to reflect a complex interaction of difficulties of auditory, verbal, visual, and gestural processing.

The present study therefore used only the first sections of the Token Test, which require the subject simply to point to one or two objects, so that the results should be obscured as little as possible by its requirements for gestural responses. The study addresses itself to an examination of four of the hypothesized components in the test: the abstract nature of the tokens, the grammatical status of the shape words, the test's dependency on short-term memory, and the role played in it by long-term or semantic memory, interpreted through a comparison of errors on this test of comprehension with errors in producing the same phrases.

It is reasonable to predict that substituting for the colored tokens common household objects which can be handled should lessen the difficulty of the task. Kreindler *et al.* (1971), in a modification of the Token

Test known as the Tridimensional Matrix Test, have demonstrated that aphasic subjects make fewer errors when the shapes they are asked to point to are drawn and labeled as flowers and houses rather than circles and squares. Geschwind (1965) and Gardner (1973) have proposed that the difficulty of color names for the aphasic is enhanced by the fact that colors can only be experienced through one sensory modality, vision. In Gardner's experiment "operativity" had a significant effect on aphasics' ability to name objects—operative objects being defined as those which are discrete and "lend themselves to manipulation, transformation and have appeal to multisensory modalities [p. 218]." One possible complication in the prediction is that the color names used in the Token Test are of higher frequency in the language than are the names of most materials. Gardner, however, was able to show that operativity was more influential than word frequency in his task.

Using materials rather than colored tokens for parallel versions of the Token Test also offers an opportunity to examine some linguistic aspects of the test. By selecting from a limited set of words for materials in common use, it is possible to keep morphophonemic form constant while changing grammatical class and denotation. For example, the words *tin* and *square* can be combined so that either can take the nominative role or the adjectival role, as in "tin square" and "square tin." In this case the referents are different: A tin square would be expected to be a flat piece of metal, while a square tin would be expected to be a container. In adjectival use, words for materials have no implications of shape, but relate to mass substance. In nominative use, however, they can function as count nouns rather than mass nouns, and have implications of shape, structure, and operativity. By careful choice, words can be found which, when paired with "square" in either order, keep the same referent, for example, "the cloth square," "the square cloth," even though one may be more probable than the other as a description of the same object. Two parallel versions of a test can therefore be produced, with the material and shape names in the same order as the color and shape names in the Token Test in one version, and in the opposite order in the other. While both use the same referents and therefore the same visual display, with the same morphophonemic form of the words, one retains the abstract token nature of the original test, despite the addition of multisensory associations (cf. "the cloth square" and "the yellow square"), while in the other tokens have become things ("the square cloth"). Differences in the number of errors produced by aphasic subjects on such parallel forms must be attributable to linguistic factors such as plausibility of usage, the count–mass reversal, the token–thing distinction. They cannot be attributed to mnestic elements in retaining auditory information as such, or in scanning a display, nor can they be attributed to praxic elements in the gestural responses required.

However, within the series of instructions in the Token Test, as well as in such parallel multisensory versions, there is scope for distinguishing mnestic influences. The test sentences increase in the amount of information they contain from the initial one-word screening section to two substantive words in Part I (e.g., "yellow square"), to three in Part II (e.g., "large yellow square"), to four in Part III (e.g., "yellow square and green circle"), to six in Part IV (e.g., "large yellow square and small green circle"). Aphasic patients are claimed to be deficient in auditory–verbal short-term memory (Albert, 1976). Therefore, if the overriding influence on their errors on the Token Test is the amount of information to be retained, then we should expect the number of errors to rise in direct proportion to the amount of information to be acted on. This should be the case regardless of the version of the test to be used. Moreover, with a deficit in short-term memory in aphasia, the "recency effect" of superior recall of final items is reported to be absent (Saffran & Marin, 1975). We should therefore predict fewer errors within each sentence on its earlier items than on its later items (the "primacy effect" of long-term memory), particularly if the items were ones which aphasic subjects could rehearse (Locke & Deck, 1978). Furthermore, if coping with recall of order as well as with recall of items were to be a significant factor in the patients' difficulties, we should expect some amalgamations in responses. Some patients would point to one item instead of to two, combining elements of both labels in the one response.

The extent to which such mnestic difficulties are dependent upon input (short-term auditory–verbal memory) or are a reflection of a more central impairment in retrieval from long-term or semantic memory can also be illuminated by comparing aphasic subjects' performances on these comprehension tests with their utterances of test items. A particularly sensitive index of difficulty seems to be aphasics' abilities to reconstitute, for speech or for comprehension, phrases consisting of adjective + adjective + noun. Lesser (1976) found that 82% of her sample of aphasic subjects made errors when asked to identify a token from such a phrase, even though 79% of these could identify more units as sequences of named objects. Gleason, Goodglass, Green, Ackerman, and Hyde (1975) reported this grammatical construction as one of the most difficult for Broca's aphasics to produce in their Story Completion Test. Scolaro and Flowers (1977) have also commented that "the task of processing sequences of three elements [size, color, shape] may have exceeded the ability [p. 6]" of the subjects they used to examine the effect of varying the pauses within or between Token Test commands. They found that lengthening the pauses did not improve performance in Part IV of the test, although it did in Part III. Since Shallice and Butterworth (1977) have argued that spontaneous speech does not use the auditory–verbal short-term memory system (on which language comprehension is partly dependent), if significant correlations are found between the comprehension and production of such phrases, the inference must be that any explanation of the diagnostic efficiency of the Token Test in terms of mnestic deficits must include impairment of processing capacity in semantic memory as well as short-term memory.

The present study therefore used the initial sections of the Token Test (the screening section plus Parts I–IV) in the version used by Spreen and Benton (1969), together with two parallel versions with words for materials substituted for those for colors. These two versions differed in the order of shape and material words. A control group of subjects was used in order to establish the degree of plausibility of the labels for the items. Aphasic subjects were also asked to describe four of the tokens and objects used in each test, and to repeat heard descriptions of them. The hypotheses tested were:

1. That the versions using objects with multisensory associations would result in fewer errors.
2. That despite the control of all other variables, the differences of grammatical class of the material and shape words in the two multisensory versions would have a significant effect on the number of errors, and specifically that the version referring to things would produce fewer errors than the version referring to tokens.
3. That the number of errors would increase with item length, and that a primacy effect of order would be found, together with amalgamations.
4. That errors of comprehension would correlate with deficits in the ability to reconstitute three-word syntagms in speech.

## SUBJECTS

The 24 aphasic subjects, 15 men and 9 women, had all suffered vascular accidents; in 23 of them these were idiopathic strokes of thrombo-embolic or intracerebral hemorrhagic origin, while the remaining subject had suffered damage to the left cerebral hemisphere following severing of the left common carotid artery in a pub brawl. The mean age was 55.67 years (range 24–73). All but 5 had left school at the minimum age of 14 or 15. All were at least 3 months post-ictus (range 3–73, mean 18.75). Fifteen were hemiplegic. On the Boston Diagnostic Aphasia Examination (Goodglass & Kaplan, 1972), 8 subjects were rated at a severity level of 1; 6 at a level of 2; 7 at a level of 3; 2 at a level of 4; and 1 at a level of 5. Five were fluent; 12 had phonetically distorted nonfluent speech; 7 typically made self-aware phonemic paraphasias.

Thirteen relatives of patients and one friend of a patient served as a control group. There were 10 women and 4 men ranging in age from 39 to 79 years, with a mean age of 59.79.

## MATERIALS AND METHOD

For presentation of the Token Test a fixed format for the tokens was used with colors aligned in rows in a 4 × 5 matrix (from left to right: blue, white, green, yellow, red). For the two parallel versions of the test, card was substituted for red, sponge for green, rubber for white, cloth for yellow and chocolate for blue. The same format was used. The cards were folded cards, as used for greetings (large–16 cm, small–4.5 cm); the sponges were yellow bathroom synthetic sponges (11 cm, 2 cm); the cloths were pieces of yellow polishing cloth (18 cm, 5 cm); the rubbers were erasers (4.5 cm, and 2 cm); and the chocolates were a square slab of milk chocolate (7 cm), a 5.5 cm medallion of plain chocolate, and a square piece of chocolate and a chocolate drop both of about 2 cm. To facilitate recognition of large and small these objects were arranged in rows (like the tokens) of small circle, small square, large circle, and large square.

The commands for one version were exactly the same as in the Token Test, with the words for materials substituted for the color words, for example, "the sponge square" (Version E). For the other version, the order of shape and material was reversed, for example, "the square sponge" (Version R). Since "circle" does not function as an adjective, for Version R "round" was substituted rather than the low frequency word "circular," for example, "the round sponge." Since this introduced a new variable of word change, data for the "square" phrases were analyzed separately where appropriate.

Before presentation of Versions E and R, aphasic subjects were given a familiarizing period of manipulating the materials to emphasize multisensory associations, that is, they were asked to stand the cards up; to squeeze the bathroom sponges; to smell the difference between milk and plain chocolate; to rub out a pencil mark; and to feel the softness of the cloth. An example of one handling instruction is "Here is a rubber, for rubbing out pencil. Feel how it bends. Can you rub out this mark? This one is a square, a rubber square, a square made of rubber. This one is round (hand to patient), a circle made of rubber, a rubber circle. Here is a small one, a small rubber circle. And here is a small rubber square. Feel how they bend."

Immediately following the comprehension test, all but four of the materials or tokens were removed. These four were the small cloth–yellow circle, the large card–red square, the large sponge–green circle, and the small rubber–white square, as appropriate. The subject was then asked to repeat the three-word descriptions of each of these items in turn, after they were spoken by the experimenter. He was then asked to tell the examiner what each item was. If the subject was unable to do this, a standard cue was used, for example, "This is the small cloth. It is round. It is the . . .?". The subject's responses were tape recorded, as well as being transcribed at the same time to ensure a pause between items.

Each subject completed all three test sets. Orders of presentation were counterbalanced, using six groups with four members each. Allocation to group was by throw of a die. There was an interval of at least 1 week and not more than 3 weeks between one test and the next.

The control subjects were given Version E only, without the initial handling and screening sections and the repetition task. Immediately after the comprehension test, control subjects were asked what they would say if they wanted the experimenter to point to each of the four items. They were also asked to do the same for the four items from the Token Test.

A "lenient weighted scoring" (Zaidel, 1977) was used for the comprehension tests, that is, one point per unit of information correctly acted upon, giving a maximum score of 60 (8 for Part I, 12 for Part II, 16 for Part III, and 24 for Part IV). The nature of the errors was recorded, in most cases it was unambiguous. In doubtful cases the most favorable score was given; for example, if the subject would have achieved a better score by pointing to partially correct items in a different order, he was credited with this. If only one item was pointed to instead of two (e.g., if the large white square was indicated instead of the large white circle and the small green square), the score was accorded to the item which was nearer to a correct interpretation (e.g., "large" and "white" would be scored as correct, with the other four units of information scored as incorrect). One repetition of the sentence by the examiner was allowed in Part I only, but this was rarely requested.

The repetition and description tasks were scored in terms of the number and kind of omissions and semantic paraphasias. Articulatory deviancies and phonemic paraphasias where a target word could be identified were not reflected in this scoring. If a phonemic paraphasia during a series of attempts at a target word happened to be an acceptable but contextually inappropriate word (e.g., "flare" for "square"), it was not scored as a semantic paraphasia. Semantic paraphasias included: oval, thin, very tiny kind, lemon, brick, post, books, cutting, toffee, paper, ring, very soft, circumference, plus incorrect applications of the given color, size, shape, and material words. Most of these paraphasias could be related to the target categories. Since the control subjects used a number of nontarget words in their descriptions (big, little, india rubber, cardboard, and round instead of circle) these were accepted from the aphasic subjects in the description tasks. The exact word was required, however, for a correct score in the repetition tasks. On both these kinds of tasks, an omission score was recorded if there was no recognizable attempt to include that category of information, even with semantic paraphasia or phonemic paraphasia. The omission score for description was based on the best attempt before the cue was given. The score for semantic paraphasia was based on any occurrence during all attempts before or after the cue. Repetitions of the same semantic paraphasia were not scored twice. Disjointed responses and missequenced words (of which there were many) were not penalized in description, since some of the responses from the controls showed these features.

## RESULTS AND DISCUSSION

Three of the control subjects made one error in pointing to items on the Version E test, and one made two. Three errors related to "rubber," one to "card," and one to "circle." Despite their preparation by the comprehension test for describing the objects as "circle" rather than "round," they overwhelmingly used the latter in their descriptions, both in the Token Test and Version E. Only four used the exact sets of words expected. Some gave partial information first (e.g., "round yellow sponge, large," "small square, white," "small cloth, the round piece of cloth"), duplicated the shape description with "round green circle," or completed the color phrases with "one" (e.g., "big, red, square one"). In fact, considering the preparation from hearing the words in the comprehension test, the description task was surprisingly difficult for control subjects. It became clear that for most of the control subjects, the phrases of the Token Test Version E were not ones they would have spontaneously used. In particular, they were more likely to end the phrase with a word for material rather than shape, and to say "round" rather than "circle."

The results for the aphasic subjects' errors on the comprehension tests are given in Table 5.1. Two subjects made no errors on the Token Test; one subject made no errors on Version R; all subjects made errors on Version E, the minimum number of errors being four. There was no effect of order of presentation of the tests (Friedman test: $x_r^2 = 2.27$, n.s.)

Error correlations among the tests were high though there was a significant difference in difficulty among the tests. Contrary to prediction Versions E and R were not easier than the Token Test; Version E was significantly more difficult. It is difficult to account for such a result entirely in terms of the lower frequency of words for materials, since Version R was of about the same difficulty as the Token Test. A contributing factor may have been the less consistent distinction between sizes, and the greater spread of the array than in the Token Test. The control subjects' descriptions suggest that the most important influence may have been the remoteness of the labels from everyday usage, perhaps being particularly great when attached to household objects rather than to colors which are more likely to be encountered as distinguishing tokens than are materials. At all events there was no evidence at all for facilitation from multisensory associations.

For examination of the effect of grammatical class and its associated semantic changes, only the data from the phrases using "square" were used, since it was only with these that morphophonemic form was constant. Since one aphasic subject had pointed only to circles throughout Parts III and IV, only 23 subjects were used in this analysis. As there were unequal occurrences of each category of word, they were each weighted to a scale of 28. In the Token Test the order of difficulty was the same as that found by Kreindler *et al.* (1971) and Zaidel (1977) in his study of the right hemispheres of commissurotomized patients, with size easier than color which was easier than shape (see Table 5.2). The dif-

**TABLE 5.1**
*Aphasic Subjects' Errors on Comprehension* [a,b]

| Test version | Mean | Standard deviation |
|---|---|---|
| Token Test | 14.33 | 11.31 |
| Version E | 18.04 | 10.11 |
| Version R | 14.75 | 11.41 |

[a]Friedman test: $x_r^2 = 9.77$, $p < .01$.
[b]Correlation coefficients (Spearman): Token Test with Version E = .82 ($p<.001$); Token Test with version R = .84 ($p<.001$); Version E with Version R = .89 ($p<.001$).

**TABLE 5.2**
*Aphasic Subjects' Errors on Comprehension of Phrases with "Square": Effect of Word Position*[a,b]

| Test version | First word | Second word | Third word | $\chi^2$ |
|---|---|---|---|---|
| Token Test | size<br>115 | color<br>132 | square<br>158 | 6.95* |
| Version E | size<br>182 | material<br>152 | square<br>208 | 8.69* |
| Version R | size<br>154 | square<br>158 | material<br>134 | 2.22 |

[a] Two-tailed sign test (Bradley): Probability of difference between
"size" errors on Token Test and Version E:   $p<.001$
"size" errors on Token Test and Version R:   $p<.05$
"square" errors on Token Test and Version E:   $p<.02$
"square" errors on Version E and Version R:   $p<.02$
[b] $N = 23$: Errors weighted to scale of 28 maximum.
*$p<.05$.

ference among the word categories was significant between the Token Test and Version E. However, the increase in difficulty of Version E over the Token Test was not specifically in terms of more errors with words for materials than words for colors, but rather was due to a generalized spread of confusion affecting size and shape more than materials. Size was predictably more difficult with the variation introduced by the materials. Words for materials as adjectives did not result in significantly more errors than those for materials as things, but there were significantly more errors with "square" in the nominative form rather than the adjectival. Thus there was no evidence for the effect of grammatical class on the words for materials, nor was there any indication that the token–thing distinction influenced the aphasic errors as far as materials were concerned. The facilitation of square as an adjective rather than as a noun is consistent with the control subjects' use of "a square one," and corroborates De Renzi and Vignolo's (1962) observation that some of the difficulty with the Token Test may lie in the grammatical status of the shape words. Cohen *et al.* (1977) have suggested that the Token Test is not so much a test of language comprehension as of analytic and abstractive capacity. They found a significant impairment in 19 Broca's aphasics on a nonverbal version of the test. In contrast it would be difficult to account for the present results with "square" other than as reflecting specifically linguistic processing.

The relationship, in the aphasics' data, between percentage of errors and units of information to be processed gave some support for the hypothesis that deficits in short-term memory can account for some of the difficulty aphasic patients experience with the Token Test. More subjects showed an increasing percentage of errors, part by part, than a decreasing or level percentage. This difference was statistically significant in 8 out of the 12 transitions in the three tests (see Table 5.3; subjects who made no errors on a test are excluded). However, the clearest jump in difficulty occurred from Part III to Part IV, with the change from one noun phrase to two, and the new requirement to point to two objects instead of one. A relatively high proportion of subjects showed a decrease in errors when size words were added to the noun phrases to make Part IV, but some of this effect was an artifact of the large increase in errors at the previous transition. Nevertheless, there were three subjects who did not produce the largest percentage of errors

**TABLE 5.3**
*Aphasic Subjects' Errors in Comprehension: Changes in Percentage of Errors with Increasing Units of Information*

|  | Test version | | |
|---|---|---|---|
|  | Token Test ($N=22$) | Version E ($N=24$) | Version R ($N=23$) |
| Change from 1 unit to 2 (screening, 1 object) | | | |
| Increase | 9 | 13 | 12 |
| Same | 10 | 10 | 8 |
| Decrease | 3 | 1 | 3 |
| $\chi^2$ | 3.91 | 7.75* | 5.30 |
| Change from 2 units to 3 (1 object) | | | |
| Increase | 13 | 14 | 13 |
| Same | 4 | 4 | 4 |
| Decrease | 5 | 6 | 6 |
| $\chi^2$ | 6.64* | 7.00* | 5.83 |
| Change from 3 units to 4 (1 to 2 objects) | | | |
| Increase | 15 | 18 | 16 |
| Same | 2 | 1 | 3 |
| Decrease | 5 | 5 | 4 |
| $\chi^2$ | 12.64*** | 19.75*** | 13.65*** |
| Change from 4 units to 6 (2 objects) | | | |
| Increase | 12 | 12 | 15 |
| Same | 2 | 0 | 2 |
| Decrease | 8 | 12 | 6 |
| $\chi^2$ | 6.91* | 4.00 | 11.56** |

*$p < .05$.
**$p < .01$.
***$p < .001$.

in Part IV on any of the three tests, and seven who produced the largest percentage in this part on only one test. To account for the major jump in difficulty from three to four units rather than from four to six, linguistic and praxic factors must be invoked as well as mnestic; this jump occurs when two noun phrases have to be matched with gestures to two objects.

Evidence corroborating the influence of short-term memory on subjects' performance was found from analysis of Part III and Part IV responses. Twelve of the subjects failed to point to a second object on at least one sentence, eight of them showing this behavior on all the test versions. In addition, two more subjects gave no response at all to one sentence. Ten subjects showed evidence of amalgamations of phrases or perseveration of word sense from the first phrase to the second (e.g., "red square" instead of "red circle and green square," "white circle and green square" instead of "white square and green circle," or "large white square and small white square" instead of "large white square and small green circle"). However, with such amalgamations excluded (because of the difficulty of allocating such errors to one or other phrase), a comparison of errors on first and second phrases gave no clear support for a primacy effect. On Part IV there was a trend for an increase in errors on the second phrase in all the versions (Token Test 34:54; Version E 60:63; Version R 47:66) but this reached a .05 significance level only with the Token Test. The demonstration that amalgamations did occur relatively frequently suggests that the mnestic deficit may not necessarily represent a failure to store items, but rather may be a breakdown in what Aaronson (1974) has described as "very limited handling capacities between two different levels of processing [p. 129]," the sensing and the identification of verbal data. Such coding delays are particularly associated with errors of order such as the amalgamations illustrate.

Such a processing failure might be restricted to input rather than reflected in aphasics' utterances. For the analysis of utterances in this respect, omissions and semantic paraphasias were combined; since precision of semantic definition may impose more demands on the identification processor, semantic paraphasias as well as omissions could reflect overloading of limited capacity. Two subjects made unintelligible responses for the descriptions, and for the analysis they were scored as having the maximum number of omissions, 12. The repetition task, as well as the description task, proved to be difficult for the aphasic group; only five subjects made no omissions or semantic paraphasias on repetition of the three-word phrases.

Errors of comprehension and of description showed high intercorrelations, though this was less so between comprehension and repetition, which is relatively more dependent on the intactness of phonological processing (see Table 5.4). Since neither broken and agrammatic productions, nor phonemic paraphasias and phonetic distortions were penalized in the scoring, the errors in description presumably reflect a semantic breakdown, or a breakdown in an early stage of word-formation—the pairing of semantic and phonological structures, such as Poeck, Kerschensteiner, Stachowiak, and Huber (1974) have postulated occurs in anomia. The high correlations between comprehension and description found here can be interpreted as evidence for an aphasic deficit in a central semantic or semantic–phonological processor, in agreement with earlier observations of parallels between word-comprehension errors and anomia in speech (Derouesné & Lecours, 1972; Goodglass & Baker, 1976; Schuell, 1966). Table 5.5 shows the relationship of word position with the number of omissions and semantic paraphasias in description and repetition. In repetition, there was a tendency for the last word to be omitted least often, regardless of its meaning, consistent with the echoic nature of this task. In description, size was the most likely to be omitted. The production tasks showed no relationship to the comprehension tasks in respect of the categories of words, reflecting the inherently different motivations of the tasks, which did not, however, detract from the commonality of level of impairment in description and comprehension.

**TABLE 5.4**
*Aphasic Subjects' Errors on Production*[a]

| Test version | Omissions and semantic paraphasias | |
|---|---|---|
| | Mean | Standard deviation |
| Description | | |
| Token Test | 6.13 | 4.28 |
| Version E | 6.46 | 3.15 |
| Version R | 7.29 | 3.98 |
| Repetition | | |
| Token Test | 3.17 | 3.00 |
| Version E | 3.29 | 3.32 |
| Version R | 2.75 | 3.30 |

[a] Correlation coefficients (Spearman):
Token Test comprehension with description = .64 ($p<.001$)
Token Test comprehension with repetition = .25 (n.s.)
Version E comprehension with description = .80 ($p<.001$)
Version E comprehension with repetition = .42 ($p<.05$)
Version R comprehension with description = .81 ($p<.001$)
Version R comprehension with repetition = .52 ($p<.01$)

**TABLE 5.5**
*Aphasic Subjects' Errors on Production: Effect of Word Position*

| Test version | First word | Second word | Third word | $\chi^2$ |
|---|---|---|---|---|
| Description | | | | |
| Omissions[a] | | | | |
| Token Test | Size 35 | Color 16 | Shape 19 | 8.94* |
| Version E | Size 28 | Material 25 | Shape 15 | 2.09 |
| Version R | Size 35 | Shape 22 | Material 19 | 5.71 |
| Semantic paraphasias[b] | | | | |
| Token Test | Size 3 | Color 23 | Shape 22 | 15.88*** |
| Version E | Size 9 | Material 18 | Shape 25 | 7.66* |
| Version R | Size 14 | Shape 27 | Material 20 | 4.16 |
| Repetition[c] | | | | |
| Omissions | | | | |
| Token Test | Size 17 | Color 18 | Shape 10 | 2.53 |
| Version E | Size 23 | Material 26 | Shape 13 | 4.48 |
| Version R | Size 15 | Shape 16 | Material 10 | 1.51 |
| Sematic paraphasias | | | | |
| Token Test | Size 3 | Color 15 | Shape 13 | 8.00* |
| Version E | Size 2 | Material 3 | Shape 12 | 10.71** |
| Version R | Size 4 | Shape 11 | Material 10 | 3.44 |

[a] $N = 21$, excludes one subject with no errors and two subjects with unintelligible responses.
[b] Excludes unclassifiable responses.
[c] $N = 19$, excludes five subjects with no errors.
*$p < .05$.
**$p < .01$.
***$p < .001$.

## CONCLUSION

From the surprising difficulty experienced by the control group of patients' relatives in constructing three-word descriptions of shapes, one conclusion can be drawn: It must not be assumed that the patients would necessarily have had such an ability premorbidly. It was for this reason that agrammatic productions in the aphasic group were not penalized in the scoring, and that a liberal interpretation was given for semantic paraphasias. It would seem that premorbid linguistic facility can easily be overestimated, even at this apparently simple level, and that relatives and patients are not unaffected by the inhibition upon performance produced by a constrained situation.

The increase in comprehension errors in Version E which was attributed chiefly to size and shape words rather than to material words suggests that it was not only the "multisensory" material words themselves which were taxing comprehension. There seemed rather to be some general irradiation of difficulty from the situation, from which the material words themselves were relatively immune, if the scoring method really was reflecting the quality of the responses accurately. More important than multisensory associations as such would seem to be their arousal in a situation where these associations are appropriate to the task. Paradoxically enough, the use of common household objects in this formal test situation seems to have had the effect of increasing its artificiality rather than reducing it. Perhaps the normal usage of such objects distracts from the test's analytic requirements more than do colored chips which are more readily accepted as tokens. Even Version R, using descriptions which came more readily to the tongue than the phrases of the Token Test for the control subjects, was slightly more difficult for the aphasic subjects than the Token Test itself. This happened even though semantic confusions seem to be less likely between words for materials than between color words, judging from the semantic paraphasias produced in speech.

That the form of language was also influential was demonstrated in the significant facilitation of the materials version when it was presented with all variables constant except the syntactic–semantic consequences of changing word order. Even though short-term memory can be invoked to account for some aspects of the Token Test results, there are discrepancies which cannot be explained in terms of more errors with more information processing. Whatever other influences there are on Token Test results—such as can be inferred from Cohen *et al.*'s (1977) and Lesser's (1976) comparisons with nonverbal cognitive, visual, and praxic tests—syntactic–semantic deficits must play a part in the commonality between aphasic comprehension on this test and production of test phrases in speech.

Within the multidimensional nature of the Token Test, this study has confirmed the partial contributions of short-term memory, semantic memory, and grammatical influences in the test's initial sections, but it suggests that factors more important than the abstract and unisensory nature of the tokens are contextual plausibility (in its widest sense) and the artificiality of a test situation.

## ACKNOWLEDGMENT

The author gratefully acknowledges the substantial help of Judith Shuttleworth in the preparation and execution of this experiment.

# III
## NEUROLINGUISTIC ANALYSES

# 6
## Lexical, Syntactic, and Semantic Aspects of the Token Test: A Linguistic Taxonomy

HARRY A. WHITAKER AND
HAIGANOOSH WHITAKER

The original purpose and the basis for the continued popularity of the Token Test is the fact that it tests language comprehension in relative isolation from visual-spatial factors, general cognitive-intellectual abilities, nonverbal memory capacity and sociolinguistic contextual cues (De Renzi & Faglioni, 1975; De Renzi & Vignolo, 1962). The Token Test also avoids unusual syntactic constructions, rare words, and linguistic redundancies all of which contribute to its credibility and usefulness as an instrument for assessing language impairments following brain damage. A number of studies have used the Token Test (reviewed and reported in this volume) with various clinical and experimental populations; only two, however (Whitaker & Noll, 1972; Whitaker & Selnes, 1978), have discussed aspects of the linguistic structure of the test. The linguistic analysis presented in those two papers is reviewed and extended in this chapter.

The application of linguistic theories to psychological research is well established; with the recent publication of such books as Goodglass and Blumstein (1973) and Lesser (1978) such application hardly needs justification in neuropsychological research. Nevertheless, it is fair to point out that the range of possible applications has scarcely been realized. In the first place, few test instruments, the Token Test included, manipulate linguistic variables in a systematic manner; second, no neuropsychological test in current use begins to approach the array of linguistic facts that are readily obtained from any recent linguistics or psycholinguistics text. It is our hope that this situation will noticeably change in the very near future.

It has been well known for many years that word frequency, the average number of times that a particular word appears in actual language use, has a measurable effect on linguistic performance. For the English language, the standard reference for word frequency data used to be Thorndike and Lorge (1944); however, this reference work has been superseded by Kuçera and Francis (1967), which is not only more current but usefully organized for statistical purposes. Considering the content words used in the various forms of the Token Test (the nouns, verbs, adjectives, and adverbs), the Thorndike and Lorge rating classifies all of them as AA (over 100 occurrences per million words), except *rectangle* (5 per million) and *slowly* (rated A, more than 50 but less than 100 per million). The function words used in the Token Test are also all rated at AA by Thorndike and Lorge, except for *underneath*, which is rated at 21 per million.

The Kuçera and Francis data give a more precise frequency count for each word, and its exact rank order, which provide a better basis for evaluating word frequency effects in the Token Test. Each word in the Kuçera and Francis primary table is given three numbers: The first number is the total number of times that the word appeared in the entire corpus of 1,014,232 words sampled; the second number indicates the number of genres, or writing styles, the word appeared in out of a total of 15 different genres (newspapers, fiction, and nonfiction, etc.); and the third is the number of 2000-word samples into which the total corpus was divided out of a total of 500 such samples. In other words, the data for the word *touch* is 87-15-062, which means that the word appeared 87 times out of a million+ words, was found in all 15 of the different genres samples, and appeared in 62 of the 500 different 2000 word samples the corpus was divided into. From this data, Kuçera and Francis constructed a rank-order table. The rank of the word *touch* is No. 1,224th (the word *the* is the most frequent word in the corpus, having the rank of No. 1). Listed in Tables 6.1–6.3 are the Kuçera and Francis frequency values for all of the words used in the various English forms of the Token Test. For convenience in referring to these tables, the words are divided into form classes, and within each form class, the words are rank-ordered with the most frequent listed first and the least frequent listed last.

Consider first the function words. As is generally known, the closed sets of function words (articles, auxiliaries, conjunctions, prepositions, pronouns) are among the most frequently used words in English. With the exception of *beside* and *underneath,* the function words used in the

**TABLE 6.1**
*Function Words*

| Word | K & F data summary | Rank |
|---|---|---|
| the | 69971-15-500 | 1 |
| of | 36411-15-500 | 2 |
| and | 28852-15-500 | 3 |
| a | 23237-15-500 | 5 |
| in | 21341-15-500 | 6 |
| is | 10099-15-485 | 8 |
| with | 7289-15-500 | 13 |
| on | 6742-15-500 | 16 |
| I | 5173-15-338 | 20 |
| from | 4369-15-500 | 26 |
| or | 4207-15-492 | 27 |
| one | 3292-15-496 | 32 |
| you | 3286-15-297 | 33 |
| there | 2724-15-467 | 38 |
| when | 2331-15-468 | 45 |
| no | 2201-15-469 | 49 |
| if | 2199-15-453 | 50 |
| up | 1895-15-430 | 55 |
| after | 1070-15-378 | 86 |
| before | 1016-15-383 | 90 |
| your | 923-15-203 | 111 |
| between | 730-15-316 | 125 |
| under | 707-15-334 | 130 |
| without | 583-15-312 | 159 |
| away | 456-15-242 | 190 |
| together | 267-15-192 | 352 |
| front | 221-15-122 | 422 |
| top | 204-15-128 | 461 |
| except | 181-15-137 | 532 |
| instead | 173-15-138 | 563 |
| beside | 78-11-055 | 1376 |
| underneath | 11-06-009 | 7422 |

Token Test all occur within the 1000 most frequent words in the language. The 2 commands in Part V of the Token Test which use these 2 locative prepositions were in the middle range of difficulty for a group of children, reported on in Whitaker and Noll (1972). The command using *underneath* was the 12th most difficult and the command using *beside* was the 13th most difficult, even though they are among the shortest sentences in that part of the test:

    42. *Put the white square underneath the yellow circle.*
    53. *Put the green square beside the red circle.*

**TABLE 6.2**
*Adjectives and Adverbs*

| Word | K & F data summary | Rank |
|---|---|---|
| little | 831-15-324 | 111 |
| small | 542-15-243 | 166 |
| large | 361-15-214 | 260 |
| big | 360-15-182 | 262 |
| slowly | 115-13-078 | 904 |
| quickly | 89-14-071 | 1189 |
| white | 365-14-156 | 257 |
| red | 197-15-101 | 482 |
| blue | 143-14-085 | 697 |
| green | 116-13-077 | 897 |
| yellow | 55-12-041 | 2007 |

Both of these commands are more difficult than, for example, the complex sentence employing "if—then" conjunction:

49. *If there is a black circle, (then) pick up the red square.*

And, as might be expected, sentence #42 and #53 are more difficult than the commands which use the locative prepositions *on top of*, and *under*, by a substantial margin:

41. *Put the red circle on top of the green square.*

61. *Put the blue circle under the white square.*

There is nothing exceptional to note about the frequency distribution of the adjectives and adverbs; *quickly* is rated the 1189th most fre-

**TABLE 6.3**
*Nouns and Verbs*

| Word | K & F data summary | Rank |
|---|---|---|
| square | 143-15-070 | 697 |
| circle | 60-10-040 | 1829 |
| rectangle | 4-02-003 | 14219 |
| take | 611-15-297 | 151 |
| put | 437-15-251 | 198 |
| show | 287-15-190 | 320 |
| move | 171-14-121 | 577 |
| touch | 87-15-062 | 1224 |
| pick up | 3-02-002 | 16684 |
| using | 145-15-095 | 684 |

quent word in the Kuçera and Francis data and the others are well under the 1000 mark, except for *yellow* which is ranked 2007th. Looking at the distribution of errors in the Whitaker and Noll (1972) data with respect to color adjectives, there is a very slight tendency for those commands which include *yellow* (square or circle) to have a higher number of errors. We suspect that with the simple colors used in the Token Test it is unlikely that an effect due to the lower frequency of occurrence of *yellow* could be separated out from the other factors which influence performance.

The two nouns which characterize the tokens, *circle* and *square* are potentially of interest if one uses a version of the Token Test that has *rectangle* instead of *square*, in view of the fact that *rectangle* is a relatively low frequency word (4 occurrences in the one million plus words of the Kuçera and Francis corpus). Using a Token Test with *rectangle* in it rather than *square*, clearly challenges De Renzi and Vignolo's original notion to devise a test that did not make use of rare words, if one is administering the test to speakers of American English. The verbs, the core of the propositional structure of the commands, present an interesting picture with respect to word frequency. Except for the Verb + Particle combination, *pick up*, the most used verb in the Token Test is the rarest of the group of commonly found verbs. *Touch* is used exclusively in Parts I–IV of the Token Test and the remaining verbs are introduced in Part V. Four of these newly introduced verbs are actually more common than *touch*, although as we will presently discuss, they are more complex syntactically and semantically. Nevertheless, except for *pick up* which appears to be relatively infrequently used the other verbs are among the more common words in English. Therefore, higher error scores on commands employing these verbs would have to be accounted for by some principle other than word frequency.

Syntactically, Parts I–IV of the Token Test are unremarkable; all commands in these sections are imperative sentences employing the verb *touch*. Complexity in these sections is achieved by varying the adjectival content of the object noun phrases as well as by altering the object noun phrase from a single one to a compound one:

    1. *Touch the red circle.*

  40. *Touch the little white square and the big red square.*

In the versions of the Token Test that we have been using, not all of the possible adjectival contrasts are employed. For example, in Sentence #40 just cited, shape is held constant while size and color are contrasted. In Sentence #31, all three adjectives contrast; in Sentence #36, size is held constant while color and shape are contrasted. In this version there are no commands which hold color constant and contrast size and shape, and in no version of the Token Test with which we are aware, is there a balanced number of commands which systematically examine shape, size, and color in Imperative sentences. Shape, size, and color are, of course, examined independently as part of the pre-test screening. Therefore, while it is possible to roughly estimate short-term verbal memory problems as the subject progresses from Part I through Part IV, it is not possible to determine whether color, size, and shape contribute equally to short-term verbal memory load.

Part V of the Token Test introduces most of the syntactic and semantic variety of this test. In addition to Imperative sentences, sentences with subordinate clauses (*when, if . . . then, after, before, except for, instead of, together with, without*), adverbs (*slowly, quickly,*) and locative prepositional phrases (*on top of, underneath, away from, in front of, beside, between, under*) are introduced. In some of these, the two clauses have both verbs expressed in the surface structure:

52. *When I touch the green circle, you take the white square.*

And in others the second verb is deleted by common conditions for ellipsis:

56. *Except for the green one, touch the circles.*

Sentence #56 also illustrates the occasional use of pronominalization in the commands of Part V, in this case requiring a slightly increased verbal memory load in that the antecedent actually follows the pronoun *one* in the surface structure, in contrast with the easier-to-process "forward" pronominalization:

50. *Pick up the squares, except the yellow one.*

Sentence #52 also illustrates the one example of the overt representation of the implicit 2nd person pronoun, *you*, in all Imperative sentences.

In a spatial array there is a well known ambiguity of reference for such locative pronouns as *on top of, underneath, in front of,* and *under,* and there is a vagueness of reference for such pronouns as *away from* and *beside.* We would note, too, that there is a structural linguistic ambiguity in the prepositional phrases introduced by *with:*

43. *Touch the blue circle with the red square.*

The *with* phrase can be Instrumental (one should use the red square and touch it to the blue circle), a Reduced Relative Clause of Attribute (if it existed in the token array, one would touch the blue circle that has a red square drawn or colored in the circle), or Comitative (one would touch the blue circle and the red square concomitantly). The last interpretation, the Comitative, has at least two realizations which will be discussed below.

The linguistic information in the commands of the Token Test cannot be calculated simply by counting content words, even though it appears that the increase in content words from 3 in Part I, to 4 in Part II, to 5 in Part III, to 7 in Part IV. positively varies with the number of errors. The problem is that coordinate structures make different demands on verbal memory than the hierarchically organized attributive structures. Thus it is possible, as we discovered in one administration of the Token Test, for

27. *Touch the blue square and the white circle.*

to cause fewer errors than

12. *Touch the big green circle.*

As we have noted in studying aphasic language performance, some brain-damaged subjects find attributive, relativized material harder to process than coordinate material, and others find the opposite to be the case (Whitaker & Whitaker, 1972). The coordinate structures underlying Sentence #27 are:

(1) *Touch the square*

(2) *Touch the circle*

and the attribute structures are:

(3) *The square is blue*

(4) *The circle is white*

The more elaborate syntactic structures found in Part V have hardly been studied with respect to the demands on short-term verbal memory. As far as we know, it is not known whether manner adverbs like *slowly,* or locative phrases like *under the white square,* behave like coordinate or attributive structures. The same must be said for the deleted material in elliptical structures and the pronouns. Of course, these problems do not detract from the usefulness of the Token Test in assessing minimal language impairments; they do, however, suggest several lines of research in which further testing, using the token array of the Token Test, might proceed to elucidate these linguistic variables.

At least one of the strategies for sentence comprehension is based on an analysis of the verb, and one of the more plausible hypotheses about how a language user accomplishes that analysis focuses on the arguments (case structure) of the verb (Clark & Clark, 1977). Case grammar has some distinct advantages over standard transformational generative grammar (Stockwell, Schachter, & Partee, 1973) in that it provides a natural way of relating the common semantic elements and diverse syntactic forms of sentence groups like the following:

(5)  *Touch the square.*

*Max touched the square.*

*The square was touched.*

*Max touched the square with his thumb, etc.*

and it also provides a natural way of comparing the common elements among sentences which contain different verbs, as is true of Part V of the Token Test. As an illustration, consider the following two sentences:

(6)  *Max sent the letter to Hortense.*
(7)  *Hortense received the letter from Max.*

Clearly the "Agent" who initiated the transmission of the letter, is Max in both examples, and the "Dative" who was the recipient of the letter, is Hortense in both examples. We would then characterize the difference between the verbs *send* and *receive* as follows: *send* takes the Agent as surface subject in the active and *receive* takes the Dative as surface subject in the active. We also note that *send* allows a passive form in which either the Dative or the Objective (*letter*) is in the surface subject position, but *receive* only permits the Objective to be subject in the passive:

(8)  *\*Max was received the letter to Hortense*

(the asterisk indicates a sentence is unacceptable in English). In some case grammar analyses, few cases are used; for example, in the Stockwell *et al.* (1973) grammar, only five cases are used: Agent, Dative, Neutral, Locative, and Instrumental. A sixth case, Essive, is restricted to predicate nominals. In our analysis here we have extended the list of cases for English (as can be found in other case grammars in the linguistics literature) for the purpose of providing a more comprehensive analysis of the verbs in the Token Test. Although some liberties with linguistic formalism have been taken, the psycholinguistic utility is of more immediate concern. The cases, with examples, are given here:

(9)  *Agentive*    (AGT)    (The animate initiator of action)
*Max picked up the square.*
AGT            NEUT

*Dative* (DAT) (The animate recipient of action, or the experiencer)

*Max gave the square to Hortense.*
AGT      NEUT   DAT

*Neutral* (NEUT) (The object, or the case most closely associated with the verb)

*Locative* (LOC) (Indicates the place where action occurs)

*Put the circle under the square.*
     NEUT      LOC

*Instrumental* (INS) (Indicates what was used to accomplish the act)

*Touch the square with your little finger.*
   NEUT        INS

*Comitative* (COM) (Indicates accompaniment, being together at the same time and doing the action together).

*Together with the yellow circle, take the blue circle.*
       COM      NEUT

*Manner* (MAN) (Indicates the manner in which action was done)

*Touch the squares slowly and the circles quickly.*
   NEUT MAN     NEUT MAN

In addition to these cases (not an exhaustive list) it is necessary to add the concepts of SOURCE (S) and GOAL (G), as secondary properties of cases for certain action verbs. Source and Goal indicate the direction of either the expressed or implied action, as seen in this example:

(10)    *Take the blue circle from the table and put it in your pocket.*
         NEUT     $LOC_S$    NEUT     $LOC_G$

Source and Goal may be secondary properties of other cases as well; in the examples (6) and (7), the Agent is also the Source and the Dative is also the Goal, with respect to the transmission of the letter.

As was apparent from (5), the same verb may participate in a variety of surface sentence structures, that is, some of the cases may be obligatory and others may be optional. For example, any verb which may appear in the Imperative structure (including all the verbs of the Token Test) clearly has an optional Agent case which is deleted in this form. It happens that the action verbs of the Token Test all take a Neutral case (this is either *circle* or *square* or both) and this case is obligatory; failure to express the Neutral case after *touch, pick up,* etc., would result in an ungrammatical sentence, as can be readily determined by deleting references to *circle* or *square* in the Token Test commands.

In examining the semantic and syntactic properties of the verbs used in the Token Test, it might be useful first to indicate what they have in common. All of the verbs are +Transitive, that is, they allow the occurrence of both the Agentive and the Neutral cases:

(11)              Max touched the square.
                  AGT           NEUT

(Note that *show* and *put* require additional cases but they, too, permit the Agentive and Neutral cases. These two verbs will be discussed later.) All of the verbs used in the Token Test may occur in the Imperative and in the Passive sentence form:

(12)     The square was picked up by Max.     (Passive)

         Take the square.    (Imperative)

All of the verbs will permit the occurrence of Manner, Temporal, Instrumental, and Comitative cases (to be discussed in more detail):

(13)    Max moved the square slowly with his thumb a few minutes ago.
        AGT       NEUT  MAN         INS            TEMP

        Max put the square under the circle.
        AGT     NEUT        LOC

        Max and Hortense picked up the square together.
        AGT     COM                NEUT

        (cf. *Max picked up the square with Hortense*)

The previous observations partly define the semantic class of verbs which involve the manipulation or movement of objects; there are many other verbs in this general semantic class, although clearly not all of them would be appropriate in a testing situation: *drop, throw, lift, arrange, push, raise, set, place, slide,* etc. As an aside, one wonders whether or not a brain-damaged subject might know the general semantic class but not all of the particular or specific verb representatives. It would not be difficult to modify the administration of the Token Test in order to explore this possibility.

We have seen at least one version of the Token Test in English in which the verb *show* appeared. *Show* turns out to be a rather unusual verb, compared to the others in the Token Test; it clearly is at the fringe of this semantic class of motion verbs, if indeed it belongs to the class at all. In the first place, although an Instrumental case can be used with *show,* it is typically not a body part unlike the Instrumental associated with the other verbs.

(14)          *Show me the square.*
                      DAT  NEUT

                *The square was shown.*
                      NEUT

                *Show me those slides with the new projector.*
                      DAT    NEUT        INS

The motion-class verbs of the Token Test do not permit a sentential complement but *show* does;

(15)          *Show (me) that you can find the red circle.*
                **touch that you can find the red circle*

The deletion of the Dative in (15) strikes us a bit odd; it is probably an ellipsis that is only permitted in a highly constrained context, in the same manner as "Yes, I will" can only have a specific meaning if the hearer knows what the speaker was referring to. Therefore, we would argue that *show* requires both the Neutral and the Dative cases in its minimal surface structure representation (except in the passive structure) which makes it somewhat different from the other verbs in the Token Test [see (14)].

Seven of the 22 commands in Part V in the version of the Token Test which we have used, employ the verb *put.* It, too, has some unusual syntactic and semantic properties even though it is more naturally a member of the semantic class of verbs which involve manipulation or movement of objects. *Put* is the only two-argument (cases) verb in the whole group, that is, it is the only verb of this group which cannot appear in any surface structure without at least two cases; note:

(16)          **the square was put*
                *the square was shown*
                **put the circle*
                *touch the circle*

What is missing from the ungrammatical sentences in (16) is the Locative case; *put* requires the Neutral and the Locative cases, minimally, in its surface structure representation:

(17)          *Put the square on the circle*
                      NEUT     LOC

If cases were "additive" psychologically, one might expect the sentences which use *put* to be more difficult to process. This does not appear to be true; in the Whitaker and Noll data, there is no evidence that *put*-sentences are noticeably difficult as all were below the mean number of errors made by the subjects in that study. There is always the possibility that different cases make different psychological demands. For example, it may be that Locative does not make the same demands on cognitive processing as Instrumental. This would account for the fact that the following *touch*-sentence incurred more errors than the following *put*-sentence:

(18)   *Touch the white circle without using your right hand.*
       *Put the green square away from the yellow square.*

However, there are other explanations, one of which is discussed here. In any event, Stockwell *et al.* (1973) argue on linguistic grounds that the cases should be systematically ordered after each verb, the overall order of all the cases for English being the same no matter what the verb. It would indeed be of interest if it could be shown that there was a psychological order to the cases, too, such that some cases were more prominent cognitively and others were less so.

In the following analyses of the case structure of each of the verbs used in the Token Test, we will omit references to the Temporal case, which specifies the time of the action, and the Benefactive case, which specifies for whom or for what the action was done. In the usual testing situation, both of these cases are pretty much implicit: A subject is carrying out the test items "on behalf of" the interviewer and the time-of-occurrence is immediate. In one of the Token Test commands, Sentence #52, the potential use of the Temporal case is exploited in the form of a temporal adverbial clause:

52. *When I touch the green circle, you take the white square.*

and the interviewer is instructed to wait about 5 sec before touching the green circle. Our analyses will use the cases listed in (9).

The case frame for *touch* is given in (19); all of the cases except Neutral are optional, that is, only the Neutral case is required in the surface structure as was noted before. Optional cases are indicated by parentheses.

(19)  *Touch:*  (AGT)   NEUT   (INS)   (COM)   (MAN)

One of the interesting features of *touch*, as noted in Whitaker and Noll (1972) and Whitaker and Selnes (1978) is that it appears to have an implicit instrumental associated with its basic lexical meaning. When not overtly specified in the surface structure, *touch* implies that one uses a body part to do the touching with and further, that the body part is usually a finger of the preferred hand. Consequently, when negating the implicit instrumental, one finds a command like Sentence #51 of the Token Test:

> 51. *Touch the white circle without using your right hand.*

As an aside, note that the Instrumental case and a clause constructed with the verb *use*, are alternative ways to say the same thing:

(20)     *Write down the answers with a pencil.*
         *Use a pencil to write down the answers.*

The exact linguistic structure of these sentence types need not concern us here, other than to note that the *use*-clause should be considered an Instrumental case. The preposition *with* is the typical marker of Instrumental case; however, it is also used to mark the Comitative case and in a limited structure, the special use of Neutral case in possessives (derived from a relative clause).

(21)     *Max went to the movies with Hortense.*
         AGT           LOC          COM

         *Max and Hortense went to the movies.*
         AGT     COM                LOC

         *Max bought a car with a red top.*
         AGT           NEUT         $NEUT_{poss}$

The Comitative use of *with* is (transformationally) related to a coordinate structure with *and*; all of these case options are shown in (21). The Comitative and the straight coordinate are not always easy to separate; we have interviewed speakers who are able to interpret Sentence #43 as shown:

43. *Touch the blue circle with the red square.*

    MEANINGS:  1. *Touch the blue circle which has a red square marked on it.*
                                2. *Use the red square as an instrument for touching the blue circle.*
                                3. *Touch the blue circle and the red square at the same time.*

In view of these possibilities, and in view of the fact that Parts I–IV of the Token Test use the verb *touch* with single and ordinary conjoined Neutral cases (object NPs), it is hardly surprising to find that Sentence #43 creates a special difficulty for subjects.

Another way of looking at the implicit Instrumental associated with the semantic representation of *touch*, is to compare how Instrumentals may be negated in a range of verbs:

(22)  *listen to the radio, but don't use your ear*
*pick up the token, but don't use your hand*
*touch the token, but don't use your finger*
*move the token, but don't use the pencil*

*Listen* not only has an implicit Instrumental, one's ear, but that Instrumental cannot be negated as noted in (22); both *pick up* and *touch* have implicit Instrumental which can be negated. *Move* does not really have an implicit Instrumental, other than in the vaguest sense common to this class of motion verbs; it may have an overt Instrumental, which of course can be negated as shown. We suggest that these facts argue for a 4-level hierarchy of the degree of instrinsicality of the Instrumental case, as shown in (23).

(23) *Scale of Instrumental Intrinsicality*

| LISTEN: | (ear) | cannot negate the implicit INS | Level I |
| TOUCH: | (finger, etc.) | can negate the implicit INS | Level II |
| PICK UP: | (hand, etc.) | can negate the implicit INS | |
| TAKE: | (unspecified) | can negate the overt INS | |
| PUT: | (unspecified) | can negate the overt INS | Level III |
| MOVE: | (unspecified) | can negate the overt INS | |
| SHOW: | (? not body part) | can negate the overt INS | Level IV |

The case frames for *pick up* and *move* are the same as for *touch*:

(24) MOVE: (AGT) NEUT (INS) (COM) (MAN)
PICK UP: (AGT) NEUT (INS) (COM) (MAN)

However, there are at least two respects in which these verbs differ from *touch*. In the first place, the Comitative case for *pick up* is a much more plausible interpretation for commands analogous to those in the Token Test. For example, if there were a command like (25),

(25)  *Pick up the square with the circle.*

it is unlikely that the subject would interpret this as Instrumental; and, assuming that the tokens were of a uniform color, it would also be unlikely that such a command would be interpreted in the relative clause-possessive form. In sum, the likely interpretation is Comitative. It is interesting to note, though, how easily an Instrumental interpretation becomes the more favored one:

(26)   *Pick up the square with the two circles.*

With respect to the features Source and Goal, *touch* and *pick up* also differ insofar as the direction of action is towards or away from the subject. One would presume that for *touch* both the Neutral and the Locative cases would have the feature Goal, while for *pick up* these two cases would have the feature *Source*. *Move,* however, allows a Locative in which both Source and Goal are expressed, with correspondingly different prepositions:

(27)   *Move the red square from the left side to the right side.*
              NEUT         LOC$_S$        LOC$_G$

One other fact about *move* should be noted; it may appear in surface structure with only the Agentive case, as in the sentence "Max moved."

The case frame for the verb *take* is given in (28):

(28)
TAKE: (AGT) (DAT) NEUT (LOC) (INS) (COM) (MAN)

Note that *take* permits the Dative case and that the Dative appears to interact with and partially overlap with both the Locative and the Benefative (BEN):

(29)
*Take the carton to Max for Hortense*
     NEUT   DAT   BEN
            LOC

*Take the package for Max (for Hortense?)*
     NEUT    DAT
             BEN

*Take the laundry to the cleaners to Max* (note: assume Max is at the cleaners)
     NEUT       LOC        DAT

*Take the book to Max.*    *Take Max the Book.* (Dative movement rule)
     NEUT DAT
          LOC

The reason that these examples seem to be ambiguous is that the preposition *to* can mark the Locative and the Dative (as well as Temporal); the preposition *for* can mark both Dative and Benefactive. The appropriate context would presumably indicate to a listener which meaning was intended. *Take* permits both a Source and a Goal type of Locative. It should also be noted that both Dative and Locative have the feature Goal, for the verb *take*, when marked with the preposition *to*. *Take* may also have a Locative marked with the preposition *from,* in which case it has the feature Source.

The case frame for the verb *put* is given in (30).

(30)
PUT:    (AGT)    NEUT    LOC    (INS)    (COM)    (MAN)

As noted before, *put* is more complex in that it requires two cases in its surface structure, the Neutral and the Locative. The Locative case has the feature Goal associated with it:

(31)        *The small package was put on the counter.*
                    NEUT                LOC$_G$

In other respects, *put* does not appear to have any unusual semantic-syntactic properties.

The case frame for the verb *show* is given in (32):

(32)
SHOW:    (AGT)    DAT    NEUT    (INS)    (COM)    (MAN)

Like the verb *put, show* minimally requires two cases in its surface structure, the Dative and the Neutral:

(33)            *The large box was shown to Hortense.*
                        NEUT            DAT

Aside from the fact that *show* allows a sentential complement as previously noted, there do not appear to be any other unusual semantic-syntactic properties associated with it. See also Table 6.4.

One aspect of the Locative case has not been discussed in detail and that is its potential function in a relative clause as an attribute of an object, or as a prepositional phrase that functions within the whole sentence. Consider the sentence in (34):

**TABLE 6.4**
*Token Test Verbs*

| | | | Case Frames | | | | |
|---|---|---|---|---|---|---|---|
| *Touch* | (AGT) | NEUT | (INS) | (COM) | (MAN) | | |
| *Move* | (AGT) | NEUT | (INS) | (COM) | (MAN) | | |
| *Pick up* | (AGT) | NEUT | (INS) | (COM) | (MAN) | | |
| *Take* | (AGT) | (DAT) | NEUT | (LOC) | (INS) | (COM) | (MAN) |
| *Put* | (AGT) | NEUT | LOC | (INS) | (COM) | (MAN) | |
| *Show* | (AGT) | DAT | NEUT | (INS) | (COM) | (MAN) | |

(34)         *Put the box in the corner on the table.*
             NEUT    LOC         LOC$_G$

In this example, the first Locative is actually from a reduced relative clause, "which is in the corner," that modifies *box*. This is clarified by noting that, in the initial state (temporally), the box in fact is not on the table; the request is that the addressee should put it there. Insofar as the objects (Neutral case) of all of the Token Test verbs exist in some real space, all of the objects may be modified by a relative clause indicating location. Evidently, though, these verbs do not all accept the independent Locative case, at least not in common usage. Consider the examples in (35). (In order to appreciate the unacceptability, imagine that the table is in the middle of the room.):

(35)   *Put, on the table, the box in the corner.*
       *Take the box in the corner to the table.*
       *Take, to the table, the box in the corner.*
       *Move the box in the corner from the corner to the table.*
       *Move, from the corner to the table, the box in the corner.*
       \**show me the box in the corner by the table.*
       ?*show me the box in the corner over here, under the light.*
       ?*show me, over here under the light, the box in the corner.*
       \**touch the box in the corner by the table*
       \**touch, by the table, the box in the corner*
       \**pick up the box in the corner on the table*
       \**pick up, on the table, the box in the corner*

The peculiarity of the sentences with *show, touch* and *pick up*, when cooccurring with a sentential Locative, is that the Locative is supposed to locate the action or object in space and in these sentences there is an apparent spatial conflict between the two locatives. Two of the sentences with *show* seem more acceptable, hence the question marks, by virtue of the fact that the act of showing seems to be less restricted spatially than the action of the class of movement verbs. This is another instance of *show*'s uniqueness among verbs used in various forms of the Token Test.

We recognize that the preceding analyses are not complete with respect to the semantic and syntactic properties of the items used in the Token Test; these analyses are, however, sufficiently detailed to illustrate that the commands of the Token Test are linguistically complex as well as linguistically diverse. It is very likely the case that a number of these linguistic variables will affect a subject's performance on the Token

Test, but the only way to verify that claim is to develop different commands in which these variables are experimentally controlled. Hopefully, the previous analyses will provide the necessary linguistic guidelines to develop alternative Token Test commands which investigate some of these variables in isolation.

# 7

## Performance of Aphasic Patients in Visual versus Auditory Presentation of the Token Test: Demonstration of a Supramodal Deficit

KLAUS POECK AND WOLFGANG HARTJE

Ever since the Token Test has been introduced by De Renzi and Vignolo (1962) as a means of detecting aphasic disorders, the instructions have always been presented auditorily: The patient must decode the instructions spoken to him, and then carry out the required tasks by manipulating the well-known tokens. Many authors have studied the psychometric aspects of the Token Test, and in most studies problems of validation and cross-validation as well as item analysis were investigated in order to increase the power of the Token Test in discriminating between aphasic and nonaphasic brain damaged patients (Orgass & Poeck, 1966; Boller & Vignolo, 1966; Swisher & Sarno, 1969; van Dongen & van Harskamp, 1972; Hartje, Kerschensteiner, Poeck, & Orgass, 1973).

The problem as to which type of performance other than auditory comprehension is tested by the Token Test, that is, which type of deficit (or deficits) is common to most of the aphasic patients in contrast to brain damaged patients has rarely been investigated (e.g., Cohen, Kelter, Engel, List, & Stroner, 1976). It is an open question whether failure of aphasic patients in the tasks of the Token Test is mainly due to deficient processing of auditory signals. Considering that not only patients with Wernicke's and global aphasia, but also patients with amnesic and Broca's aphasia score significantly lower than brain damaged patients with-

**TABLE 7.1**
*Etiology and Age in the Four Subgroups of Aphasic Patients*

|  | Vascular | Traumatic | Other | Age |
|---|---|---|---|---|
| Amnesic $N = 12$ | 6 | 5 | 1 | 31.1 |
| Broca $N = 13$ | 11 | 2 | – | 47.1 |
| Wernicke $N = 8$ | 8 | – | – | 55.4 |
| Global $N = 15$ | 14 | 1 | – | 54.9 |
| Total $N = 48$ | 39 | 8 | 1 | 47.0 |

out aphasia, it is just as likely that the failure of aphasic patients in the Token Test is due to processing disorders in the central language system (Whitaker, 1971), independently of the nature of the input. We hypothesized that the functional deficit which causes the aphasic patients to fail in the Token Test is a supramodal rather than a unimodal (auditory) deficit. We therefore carried out an experiment in which the instructions of the Token Test were given in two modalities, once with acoustic (vocal instructions) and once with visual (written instructions) input.

## PATIENTS

The examination was based on 48 patients, unequivocally diagnosed aphasic on the basis of a standardized examination developed in our department. Etiology, age, and type of aphasia of these patients are given in Table 7.1. In the total group the age varied between 15 and 73 years (mean = 47 years, $SD$ = 16.7 years). The patients with amnesic aphasia were notably younger than the patients in all other subgroups.

Twelve patients (8 with global, 2 with amnesic, and 2 with Wernicke's aphasia) had a complete or incomplete homonymous right-sided hemianopia.

## METHODS

The Token Test was given in the conventional, vocal–auditory mode as well as the visual mode of presentation. For the visual mode the instructions were printed on cards of 15 × 21 cm. Half of the subjects were given the vocal version first, half the visual. The time allotted for reading the written instructions was limited, 10 sec for each instruction of Parts I–III, 15 sec for each instruction of Parts IV and V. The tokens remained covered until the patient indicated that he was ready to carry out the instruction. As soon as the tokens were uncovered, subjects were not allowed to read the instructions further.

## RESULTS

The first problem was whether the order of presentation (vocal mode first or visual mode first) had any influence on the subjects' performance. This was not the case. Neither in the visual nor in the vocal mode of presentation was there a difference between the performances in the first and second run (see Table 7.2).

No differences in performances were observed when the test was first given either in the vocal or visual mode. In other words, there was no modality-specific effect of transfer (see Table 7.3).

When we compared performances in the visual and vocal version of the Token Test there was no significant difference, neither for the total group nor for any one of the aphasic subgroups (see Table 7.4).

We also found a strong correlation between the performance in the two modes of presentation: Individual patients who performed well or poorly in one modality scored equally well or poorly in the other modality. The Spearman rank correlation was $r_s = .77$, $p < .01$.

An analysis of variance (4 × 2 factorial design with repeated measures) was performed to check possible differences between the performances of the aphasic subgroups or a possible interaction of type of

**TABLE 7.2**
*Comparison between the Token Test Performance in the First and Second Run with Visual and Vocal Presentation (U-Test, Two-Tailed p)[a]*

|  | Mean error score | |
| --- | --- | --- |
|  | First run | Second run |
| Visual | 24.4 | 24.9 |
| Vocal | 26.7 | 26.0 |

[a]None of the results show statistical significance at the 95% probability level.

**TABLE 7.3**
*Comparison of Token Test Performances in the Visual–Vocal and the Vocal–Visual Order of Presentation (Wilcoxon-Test, Two-Tailed p)*[a]

|  | Mode of presentation | |
| --- | --- | --- |
|  | Visual | Vocal |
| Visual–vocal | 24.4 | 26.0 |
| Vocal–visual | 24.9 | 26.7 |

[a] None of the results show statistical significance at the 95% probability level.

aphasia and mode of Token Test instructions. For this purpose, four age-matched subgroups of eight patients each were formed showing approximately equal means and variances with respect to age.

Results of this analysis showed a significant main effect of type of aphasia [$F(3, 38) = 3.56$], but no effect due to mode of Token Test instructions [$F(1, 28) = .94$] nor interaction between these two factors [$F(3, 28) = .51$] was found. Newman-Keuls tests showed that only the difference between the subgroups with amnesic and global aphasia reached the .05 level of significance.

In the visual presentation we found a positive correlation between the Token Test scores and the Performance-IQ: The lower the Performance-IQ, the more errors were made in the visual version of the Token Test ($r_s = .48$, $p < .05$). A similar correlation, however, was not found for the vocal presentation ($r_s = .20$, n.s.). Furthermore, it was

**TABLE 7.4**
*Token Test Performance in Visual and Vocal Presentation in the Four Aphasic Subgroups (Wilcoxon-Test, Two-Tailed p)*[a]

|  | Mode of presentation | |
| --- | --- | --- |
|  | Visual | Vocal |
| Amnesic | 15.7 | 16.4 |
| Broca | 22.4 | 23.7 |
| Wernicke | 24.8 | 29.4 |
| Global | 33.9 | 35.1 |
| Total | 23.9 | 26.4 |

[a] None of the results show statistical significance at the 95% probability level.

**TABLE 7.5**
*Comparison between Aphasic Patients with and without Right-Sided Hemianopia with Regard to Token Test Performance and Performance-IQ (U-Test, Two-Tailed p)*

|  | Visual field defect | |
|---|---|---|
|  | With | Without |
| Visual Token Test*** | 33.0 | 21.8 |
| Vocal Token Test** | 32.6 | 23.9 |
| Performance-IQ* | 81.4 | 90.2 |

*$p \leq .02$.
**$p \leq .05$.
***$p \leq .005$.

found that patients with right-sided hemianopia did less well than patients without VFD. This was true not only for the visual but also for the vocal presentation (Table 7.5). In addition, the table shows that patients with right-sided hemianopia had a significantly lower Performance-IQ.

There was no significant difference, however, in the Token Test performance with visual as compared to vocal presentation of the instructions: This was true for both the group of aphasics without hemianopia and the group of aphasics with right-sided hemianopia (Wilcoxon-Test, two-tailed, n.s.).

## DISCUSSION

De Renzi and Vignolo introduced the Token Test as a sensitive method for the detection of aphasic disturbances in language comprehension. Disturbances of comprehension in this connection are to be understood as disorders in comprehending spoken language. Further validation and cross-validation studies have demonstrated that the Token Test is susceptible only to a very limited extent to the unspecific influences of overall mental deterioration present in brain damaged patients. It has been demonstrated by numerous researchers that the Token Test measures a performance deficit which is specific or at least very characteristic for aphasic patients.

The validation and cross-validation studies have demonstrated that the discriminating power of the Token Test applies to Broca's aphasia as well as to Wernicke's aphasia, though quantitatively to a different degree. It is obvious that the Token Test captures a performance deficit which is common to all aphasic patients, independently of type of aphasia. It has also been shown that the Token Test indicates the degree of overall impairment in aphasia independent of the subtype.

These results raise the problem as to what kind of performance the Token Test really measures. Much of the past research on the Token Test has maintained that the disturbances in the understanding of spoken speech are common to all aphasics, to those with a frontal and to those with a temporal brain lesion; that is, the Token Test detects a disturbance in language understanding which lies at the root of the aphasic symptoms. Such a position is very close to the unitary concept of aphasia (*l'aphasie est une*) proposed by Pierre Marie.

It is equally possible, however, to hold the position that the test requires understanding for spoken language only prima facie, and that performance is, in fact, dependent on other factors, for example, verbal memory. One might even speculate that deficient performance in the Token Test in different aphasic syndromes is not necessarily due to the same type of deficit (Poeck, Kerschensteiner, & Hartje, 1972). Few experimental studies have been done so far. Cohen et al. (1976) found that Parts I–IV of the Token Test already differentiate very well between aphasic and nonaphasic patients, although in these parts of the Token Test language understanding is tested semantically and syntactically at a much less complex level than in Part V. The authors concluded that the discrimination between aphasic and nonaphasic patients was dependent on cognitive processes. They advanced the opinion that Token Test performance was not dependent on short-term memory. There was no correlation between Token Test scores and memory scores. Cohen et al. concluded that the Token Test captures a global left-hemispheric function which they described as the ability to analyze situations that superficially appear as *Ganzheiten* (whole). Cohen et al. treat the Token Test as a test which examines the ability to organize the parts of a whole, similar to the Hidden Figures Test (Gottschaldt, 1926, 1929). The efficiency of the Token Test in discriminating aphasic patients was interpreted by these authors as demonstrating a particular deficit of aphasic patients in this postulated left-hemispheric function.

Alternatively, one could consider that the Token Test examines a supramodal performance in the elaboration of linguistic material. In order to give at least a partial answer to these questions, we have designed an experiment in which the tasks of the Token Test are given not only in the conventional vocal form, but also in a visual form. It was our expectation that the aphasic patients, with the exception of global aphasics, would perform better in the visual mode of presentation than in the vocal one. This expectation was based on the clinical experience that most aphasics are much better in reading for understanding than in the understanding of spoken language. Contrary to our expectations, however, we found no significant differences neither in the performances of the total group of aphasics nor in the performances of the aphasic subgroups in the two modes of presentation (vocal versus visual).

The fact that we did not find a difference between the two modes of presentation could have been the result of a learning effect present in the second as compared to the first run. The alternating presentation would not have prevented such a learning effect. Therefore, it was necessary to evaluate statistically the eventual influence of the order of presentation. Tables 7.2 and 7.3 demonstrate clearly that there was no learning effect from the first to the second run, independently of the order of presentation: vocal-visual or visual-vocal. This finding corresponds to the practical experience that even repeated vocal presentation of the Token Test has no learning effect in aphasic patients.

When we tested the influence of the control variables on the Token Test performance we found a moderate, but statistically significant, correlation between the visual but not the vocal presentation of the Token Test and the Performance-IQ. This finding could mean that in both tasks visual performances are strongly involved. Furthermore, patients with right-sided hemianopia performed less well in both modes of presentation than patients without hemianopia. It is generally assumed that the additional presence of a visual field defect in aphasic patients indicates a larger extent of the brain lesion.

In summary, we have demonstrated that the Token Test detects the aphasic impairment in performance not only in the modality of auditory language comprehension, but also in the modality of visual language comprehension. It is obvious that the test is sensitive for a supramodal deficit in aphasic patients.

# IV
## CLINICAL APPLICATIONS

## 8

# Nondiagnostic Uses of the Token Test
AUDREY L. HOLLAND AND JANET L. WHITNEY

There is a tendency for language rehabilitation specialists to use tests as models for the development of clinical techniques. That is, after a given test has served its diagnostic function, it is a frequent occurrence for clinicians to "teach to" the areas of deficit a test has pointed out by elaborating treatment activities based on prototypical test items. Treatment of this type is based on the assumption that tests designed to isolate particular deficits consist of items which themselves are valid examples of those deficits, and practice or shaping of performance on similar items should perforce improve the presently defective behavior. No test is immune from such activities, regardless of the circular logic and unmeasured validity of these undertakings. The Token Test has generated some small share of them. The argument is that, if the Token Test is a valid measure of auditory comprehension, then Token Test-like activities should improve auditory comprehension in aphasic adults. We wish to make it clear that we are not questioning the validity of such an approach. Rather, our intent here is to explore the nondiagnostic uses to which the Token Test has been put. What follows is a summary of clinical research activities developed from the Token Test itself, and some clinical implications that seem to be suggested by them.

"Nondiagnostic" is applied in a special sense here. Instead of using the Token Test to measure subtle deficits in auditory comprehension, the measure has been used to investigate other aspects of auditory behavior. Its format has also been exploited and manipulated to train auditory comprehension. These two aspects are what, for purposes of this chapter, will be considered its "nondiagnostic" uses.

## AUDITORY PROCESSING

The Token Test, by virtue of its minimal vocabulary, gradually increasing complexity, and low redundancy, provides an appealing framework for investigating some parameters of auditory memory that might be differentially affected by aphasia. For example, if the primacy effect is operating, the aphasic patient might respond to the command, "Touch the yellow circle and the red square," by pointing appropriately to the yellow circle but missing the red square. The recency effect would produce the opposite result; that is, the patient would miss the yellow circle and correctly point to the red square.

As part of a larger study on auditory processing in aphasia, La Pointe, Horner, Liberman, and Riski (1974) analyzed Token Test failures along these two parameters, referring to primacy as "noise build-up" and to recency as "slow rise time." They also investigated three additional parameters: (a) retention deficits, in which overall poorer performance comes about as the stimulus becomes longer; (b) information capacity deficits, in which short bursts of accuracy interact with failure, thus producing a response such as touching a yellow square to the command "Touch the yellow circle and the red square"; and (c) intermittent auditory imperception—an apparently random fluctuation of successes and failures on Token Test items. La Pointe et al. suggest that, for some aphasic patients, characteristic Token Test performance corresponding to these processing patterns could be isolated. That is, one aphasic patient's errors might be consistently of the slow rise time pattern, while another's errors might be typified as occurring on the longer stimulus material, although both ultimately would have achieved the same Token Test score. While La Pointe et al. did not directly suggest any applications, knowledge of typical patterns could be useful in planning individual clinical strategies for increasing aphasic persons' auditory comprehension skills. For example, the Token Test could first be used to determine a patient's overall auditory comprehension deficit, and then further analyzed to isolate these patterns. If the aphasic patient is demonstrating a recency effect, it might be sensible to evolve a clinical strategy in which a constant initial task (i.e., "Pick up the gloves") was followed by a series of changing words ("gloves and hat," "gloves and glasses," etc.) allowing the patient to shift his auditory focus comfortably away from his strengths to the relatively weaker processing area.

It is unfortunate that La Pointe *et al.* did not relate the pattern observed to type of aphasia manifested by his patients. A compelling notion is that some such relationship could be used to explain the patterns observed in this study.

## TIME TO PROCESS INFORMATION

Another parameter of auditory processing that has been investigated using the Token Test has been that of time to process the information involved in the commands. In an effort to determine whether aphasics would profit from increased time to process, two studies have inserted pauses into the commands, and have compared unpaused versus paused performance by aphasic patients. While these two studies, one by Liles and Brookshire (1975) and the other by Salvatore (1975), present some minor discrepancies in their findings, both suggest rather conclusively that pausing of two seconds duration or longer facilitates comprehension of the commands. (In Liles & Brookshire's case, the pause value was a very long 5). Pause placement as well as pause length has been varied in these studies with apparently little differential effect. Thus, in clinical application, it would appear that the insertion of pauses in stimulus material designed to facilitate comprehension is justifiable, and further that insertion of longer pauses at constituent boundaries where short, normal pausing is most likely to occur spontaneously is also defensible. The facilitative effect appears to be a large one. In fact, in the study by Salvatore (1975), a group of aphasics who were exposed to pauses only during pre- and post-testing improved enough at post-test to match the performance of aphasics who had received a training program designed to fade pauses toward more normal prosody.

The overall rate of Token Test item presentation has also been altered in a recent study be Peck (1977), not with adults but with children with learning disabilities. Using Varispeech 2 playback equipment, she slowed the rate of presentation of Token Test-type commands to 110 words per minute and compared the slowed and normal versions for these children and for matched normal children as well. Learning-disabled children's performance improved under slowed conditions to approximate the normal performance. It seems likely that aphasic adults should show some related effect, although this research has yet to be done.

These positive effects of rate alteration, either by pausing or by overall slowing suggest that aphasics appear to profit from increased time to process auditory information. This effect is, most likely, due to accommodation in the impaired processing mechanism, although it possibly puts less strain on short-term memory as well.

Another way of increasing time to process information is by imposing a delay in the aphasic person's response. That is, following the spoken message, the patient is told or signaled to wait before responding. In a study by Yorkston, Marshall, and Butler (1977), aphasic subjects were exposed to three conditions: no imposed delay, a 5-sec and a 10-sec imposed delay of response. Using materials and commands similar to the Revised Token Test (McNeil & Prescott, 1978), they found that the aphasic patient's performance improved in a linear fashion with greater delay. This finding, however, has recently been contradicted by a study by Toppin and Brookshire (1978), who found delay effects only in Part III of the Token Test, and that increasing the delay interval resulted in deteriorated rather than more effective performance.

The clinical implications of these studies appear to be rather clear cut. Clinicians should utilize the information either by slowing the rate of their own speech, or possibly by imposing a delay of the aphasic person's response. Furthermore, this information should be demonstrated and shared with him, so that he can perhaps learn to request slowdowns from other speakers, or learn to impose the delay on himself. Family members and others in the aphasic person's environment can also be taught to alter their rate of speaking, or their expectation of an immediate response.

Salvatore's findings of the facilitative effect of pauses was part of a larger study in which he attempted to train aphasic patients to respond to shorter and shorter pause durations in Token Test commands; that is, until they were able to respond to commands at normal speed and prosody. This particular attempt to teach aphasic patients to process more rapidly was not overwhelmingly successful. However, the Token Test and Token Test-type commands furnish an extremely useful approach for developing other approaches to such training.

In another investigation, Salvatore, Strait, and Brookshire (1978) simply asked experienced and inexperienced clinicians to give the Token Test to a group of high and low functioning aphasic patients following the test's original instructions that the commands should be read by the examiner "speaking with a clear and measured voice, without any special prosodic emphasis [De Renzi & Vignolo, 1962]." The study showed that experienced clinicians used longer pauses in giving commands than did inexperienced ones. None of these pauses exceeded

1.25 sec, however. This increased pausing held true regardless of whether the patient was functioning at a higher or a lower level. In a second experiment, the same examiners were told to repeat missed items until the subject responded correctly or until it had been delivered three times. These repetitions were compared to the initial delivery rate. Four of the five examiners slowed their rate on these repetitions, thus showing a differential rate sensitivity to error responses.

It appears that experienced clinicians intuitively attempt to alter their rate of speaking with aphasics. While we would not advocate varying the delivery of Token Test commands to facilitate performance when the test is used diagnostically, it certainly appears that manipulation of pausing and rate of clinician speech in treatment has some justification as a way to improve comprehension. What remains for the clinician who has, on the basis of experience, already reached that conclusion is to learn to use pauses and rate changes sytematically—possibly initially increasing pause length and decreasing rate, and fading over time to more closely approximate normal speech—and to explain its usefulness to others involved with the aphasic person.

To summarize the material presented so far, the La Pointe et al. study looked at patterns of responding in a way that furthers our understanding of the interactive effects of short-term memory and language comprehension. This is an important theoretical question, not only for understanding aphasic comprehension, but for normal comprehension of language as well. The rest of the studies have manipulated presentation of the Token Test items, or the time between commands and responses to them, measuring the effects of such manipulation on Token Test performance itself. Such studies furnish some minimal generalizations about the physical characteristics of messages that might impede or facilitate their comprehension by aphasic adults. While the studies of time to process information are exemplary here, there are other possibilities worthy of investigation using the Token Test as well. For example, what effect does varying loudness have? Or live voice versus tape recorded commands? The "unabridged" Token Test appears to present a reliable baseline for undertakings of this sort that have a broader theoretical and clinical significance than Token Test performance itself.

## CLINICAL STUDIES

Most thoughtful clinicians use commands at some point in therapy, not only to check auditory comprehension of aphasic adults, but as the raw material for increasing auditory comprehension in their patients.

The Token Test's commands have been used in two such clinical research studies. The first, by Holland and Sonderman (1974), developed a systematic training program of items paralleling the Token Test. The program used principles of programmed instruction; that is, the training items gradually increased in complexity, and differential reinforcement for correct responding was provided immediately following each training item. A special feature of this differential reinforcement was the feedback given for incorrect responding in Parts I–IV. In these parts, aphasic subjects were not simply told that they were wrong, but the nature of their error was made explicit. That is, if the item required the patient to "Touch the large red circle and the small green square," and he touched the large green circle and the small red square, he was so informed. He was told, "No, Mr. X, you touched the large *green* circle and the small *red* square." The training program was given to 24 aphasic adults, pre-tested on the Token Test and also on four auditory comprehension subtests of the Minnesota Test for the Differential Diagnosis of Aphasia (MTDDA). Patients entered the training program for the part of the Token Test where their error rate was 50% or more. They stayed with the program until they finished, or until their program error rate reached a punishing 80%. They were then post-tested on the Token Tests and the MTDDA subtests. Some interesting generalizations obtained. The program significantly improved Token Test scores for moderately and mildly impaired aphasics, and generally produced no significant changes for initially low functioning aphasic patients. The one exception was an improvement for the youngest, traumatically injured patient, whose gain put him near the high group post-test mean. No generalization of this training to the MTDDA tests was shown. We consider two aspects of this research to be clinically important as they relate to the Token Test. The first was that prognosis for improvement was considerably better for patients who made it at least to Part IV before reaching a 50% error rate. This suggests some prognostic value of the test itself. The second was that the method, for higher functioning patients at least, was effective in modifying auditory comprehension as it is measured by the Token Test.

At the same time as this experimentation was in progress and aphasic patients in Pittsburgh were being differentially reinforced in a gradual progression program for circles and squares, aphasics in New York were working on an ingenious training procedure designed by Joyce West (1973). Pre- and post-training procedures were almost equivalent in the two studies. However, the training itself differed. Instead of circles and squares, the program substituted an array of objects and decorative items—various colored combs, yarn, pencils, forks, Easter eggs—which were trained in Token Test-like arrays with Token Test-like commands. A much longer program to administer (and probably a less boring one), West obtained from it similar significant increases in Token Test scores, which were maintained for four of her five experimental subjects over 8-9 months. This program also appeared to generalize to MTDDA subtests as well.

These studies together emphasize that, for some aphasics at least, auditory comprehension can be improved using procedures derived from the Token Test. Perhaps as important, they illustrate the fertility of the Token Test for directing clinical intervention. Although squares and rectangles appear to have been used almost synonymously, and the "Modified Token Test" has been used by some of the studies reported here, most of this clinical research has stuck rather closely to the format of the Token Test.

The general *form* of the Token Test—commands of increasing complexity and/or length to which motor responses (possibly including speech) are required—can provide the aphasia therapist with clinical approaches of even broader utility than the rather strict ones described here. A functional example, perhaps most properly a grandchild rather than a closer descendent of the Token Test, seems to furnish an appropriate conclusion.

Helping aphasic patients to develop strategies to facilitate their own comprehension has been described by one of the authors (Whitney, 1975). As part of a program to develop use of compensatory strategies in general, she proposed that aphasic patients with auditory comprehension deficits might be taught to request speakers to repeat their messages. For example, in a clinician-client dialogue, the clinician first specifically directs the patient to request a repetition: "Listen carefully. Ask me to repeat if you need to." An auditory command is then presented: for example, "Give me the brown shoes." If the patient responds inaccurately, he is again directed to request a repetition, "Ask me to say it again." Any indication from the patient that he is requesting a repetition is accepted, from "Say it again, please" to "Huh?" or a gestural signal to repeat the message. Only when the repetition has been requested does the clinician repeat the command.

Once the aphasic patient is using the strategy in response to specific direction from the clinician, the clinician may only prompt him to use it by asking "What do you need to do?" Each time the strategy is used, the patient is reinforced. Of course, accurate responses to the command are also reinforced, whether on the first presentation of the command, or after a repetition has been requested and received. This program, like others developed to improve the aphasic adult's auditory comprehension, builds upon the use of Token Test-like commands.

It has been the intent of this paper to suggest some subtle diagnostic and clinical uses of the Token Test. No attempt has been made to be exhaustive; rather, we have tried simply to be illustrative. As good clinicians add the Token Test routinely to their diagnostic procedures, many, many more uses of it should follow.

# 9
## Use of the Token Test with Children: Two Contrasting Socioeconomic Groups

J. DOUGLAS NOLL AND NORMAN J. LASS

Whenever it is expected that different populations of subjects will achieve different results on a particular clinical test instrument, it is important to obtain separate sets of normative data. We were interested in determining whether two culturally different communities would achieve similar scores on the Token Test. Specifically, how would a middle-class group of children and a group of children from economically disadvantaged families respond differentially to the Token Test?

In considering the effects of social class on language development, Adler (1973) states, "the nature of verbal interactions needs to be considered carefully since ethnicity may generate different values and mores which in turn may be reflected in different kinds of verbal stimulation models [p. 5]." There is a rather extensive body of literature which suggests that certain features of language usage do indeed vary as a function of social class (e.g., Bernstein, 1974; Deutsch, 1965). Most of the research, however, has been restricted to studies of the speech and language output of different social and/or ethnic groups. Little has been done on describing the nature of any differences in auditory verbal comprehension skills. The grammatical and lexical variants of the Token Test lend themselves very nicely to this type of sociolinguistic investigation.

## THE TOKEN TEST

The present study utilized a modification of the Token Test by Boller and Vignolo (1966). A copy of the test protocol is included in an appendix at the end of this paper. There are 20 plastic "tokens": 5 large circles, 5 small circles, 5 large squares, and 5 small squares, of 5 colors (red, blue, green, yellow, white). The large circles and squares are 1.5 in. in size, and the small circles and squares are 1 in. in size. The tokens were cut from sheets of ⅛ in. solid colored plexiglass. The tokens are placed on the table directly in front of the subject in a prearranged order. The examiner gives a series of oral commands and, in response, the subject executes a simple act with the plastic tokens.

The tasks are exactly defined with linguistic redundancy kept to an absolute minimum. The test is divided into five parts. In Parts I-IV, the commands are syntactically the same, that is, the imperative construction with either one or two noun phrase objects. The same verb, *touch*, is used in each item. There is a progressive increase in complexity from Parts I-IV in terms of the adjectival content of the various noun phrase objects. Also, Parts I and II contain only one noun phrase (e.g., "the red square" or "the big yellow circle"), whereas, Parts III and IV contain two noun phrases in each item (e.g., "the green square and the blue circle"). Part V introduces different verbs and different noun phrase structures in the predicates.

In scoring this test, each item is scored as either 1 (correct) or 0 (incorrect). Responses are scored in terms of total commands correct, and each command is worth one point. Therefore, failure to respond to any one element of information in the command is scored as an error. Each of the first four parts of the Token Test contains 10 items, and 22 items are included in Part V, resulting in a total of 62 items. Thus, the maximum score on the test is 62.

## PROCEDURE

The Token Test was administered to 252 children, 18 in each 6-month age group from 5:0 through 11:11. These children were selected from the public schools in the semirural areas surrounding Lafayette, Indiana. All children were white and would be fairly representative of a middle-class population. On the basis of school records, only those children were tested who demonstrated normal abilities on standard achievement or intelligence tests. Furthermore, no child with clinically deviant speech was included. This group of subjects hereafter will be referred to as the *standard* or *criterion* group. The detailed results of this segment of the study and a linguistic analysis of the error patterns can be found in the article by Whitaker and Noll (1972).

The Token Test was also administered to 252 children enrolled in an ESEA Title I program in Harrison County, West Virginia. The parents of these children had no formal education beyond high school, and many never completed elementary or high school. In order to be included in the program, the total annual income of the families was $3000 or less for four or more members in a family. The method of selection of these children to be used as subjects was identical to the standard or criterion group. That is, there were 18 at each of the 6-month age groups from 5:0 to 11:11. All subjects were white and tested within the average range on school achievement or intelligence test results. Likewise, no child was used if he/she exhibited clinically deviant speech. Hereafter, this group will be referred to as the *economically disadvantaged* group.

## RESULTS

Table 9.1 shows the mean scores, standard deviations, and ranges for the standard group and the economically disadvantaged group of

**TABLE 9.1**
*Means, Standard Deviations, and Ranges of Scores Obtained on the Token Test for Both Groups of Subjects at Each 6-Month Age Level*

| Age levels | Standard group | | | Economically disadvantaged group | | |
|---|---|---|---|---|---|---|
| | Mean | SD | Range | Mean | SD | Range |
| 5.0–5.5 | 41.8 | 7.6 | 30–56 | 28.4 | 4.4 | 20–35 |
| 5.6–5.11 | 45.4 | 6.7 | 32–56 | 33.3 | 1.8 | 30–37 |
| 6.0–6.5 | 46.1 | 8.2 | 31–56 | 41.0 | 8.3 | 25–53 |
| 6.6–6.11 | 49.3 | 6.5 | 38–60 | 43.3 | 9.8 | 23–60 |
| 7.0–7.5 | 52.6 | 3.9 | 43–57 | 45.1 | 11.0 | 27–62 |
| 7.6–7.11 | 55.8 | 3.1 | 48–60 | 48.3 | 9.2 | 20–62 |
| 8.0–8.5 | 54.7 | 3.6 | 47–60 | 53.1 | 5.8 | 38–58 |
| 8.6–8.11 | 55.4 | 2.9 | 51–60 | 52.3 | 6.2 | 39–59 |
| 9.0–9.5 | 55.8 | 5.0 | 44–61 | 51.6 | 6.0 | 42–61 |
| 9.6–9.11 | 58.0 | 2.5 | 53–61 | 52.8 | 4.6 | 44–60 |
| 10.0–10.5 | 56.4 | 4.1 | 47–62 | 52.3 | 5.5 | 35–59 |
| 10.6–10.11 | 58.3 | 2.3 | 53–62 | 55.4 | 4.4 | 45–61 |
| 11.0–11.5 | 58.7 | 1.7 | 55–61 | 57.8 | 3.7 | 48–62 |
| 11.6–11.11 | 59.0 | 2.2 | 55–62 | 55.7 | 3.9 | 49–62 |

subjects at 6-month age levels. Figure 9.1 depicts the mean number of correct responses on the Token Test for both groups at each age level.

As expected, for both groups of subjects, there is a pattern of increasingly correct test scores with increased age, although the curve tends to plateau at about 7.5 or 8.0 years of age with relatively little change after that point. Moreover, the scores of the older subjects are similar to those obtained from normal adults (Swisher & Sarno, 1969).

Inferential statistical analysis, consisting of a two-factor analysis of variance (Winer, 1972), was performed on the data. Results of the analysis indicate the following: (a) there are significant differences $[F(1,476) = 115.15, p < .001]$ between the Token Test scores of the standard and economically disadvantaged children in the study; (b) there are significant differences $[F(1,476) = 54.32, p < .01]$ between the different age groups investigated for both the standard and economically disad-

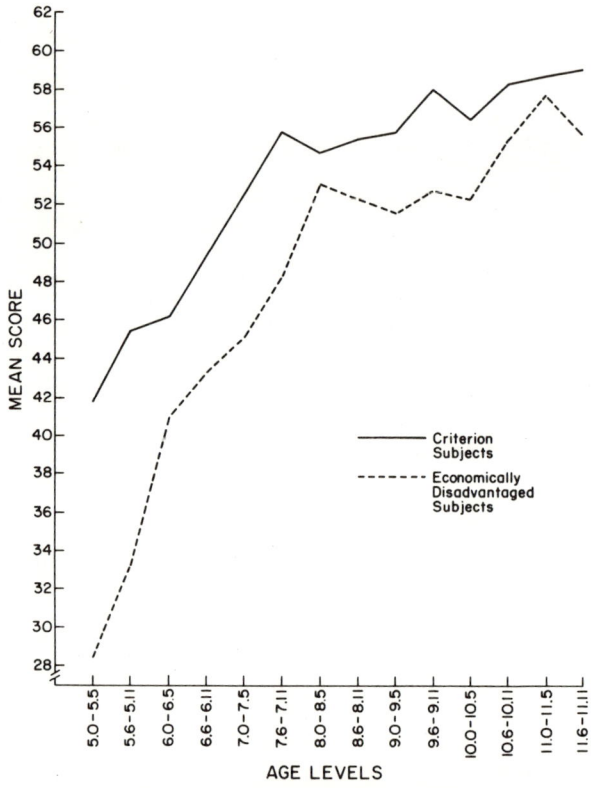

**FIGURE 9.1.** *Mean Token Test scores for the two groups of subjects and each 6-month age level.*

vantaged children; and (c) there are no significant ($F$ (1,476) = 3.62, $p > .05$] interaction effects between the factors of groups and ages of children, indicating that the Token Test scores did not vary systematically as a function of variations in age of the children and their economic group (standard versus economically disadvantaged).

In performing statistical tests (Winer, 1972) for the simple effects of the age factor to determine which age groups differed significantly from each other, it was found that children in the standard group from age 5:0 through 7:11 and from 9:0 through 10:5 showed significant differences in their Token Test scores when compared to children of the same ages in the economically disadvantaged group. There were no significant differences between the two groups for ages 8:0-8:11 and 10:6-11:11. Figure 9.1 shows that the differences between the standard and economically disadvantaged groups appear to be greatest at the younger age levels, with smaller differences occurring after age 7:11.

## DISCUSSION

The results of this study were not altogether unexpected. It simply constitutes another piece of evidence that there are social class language differences, specifically receptive language functions. It is of some interest that the differences in Token Test scores were greater at the younger ages, while at the older ages studied, the differences were nonsignificant. This is in contrast to the results obtained by Deutsch (1965). He administered a number of language tasks to 127 first grade and 165 fifth grade children representing lower-class and middle-class families. His results suggested a cumulative deficiency in language functioning, meaning that there were *greater* social class differences for the fifth grade children than the first grade children. There is no ready explanation for the difference in age–social class interaction between the Deutsch study and the present Token Test results.

One is always hard pressed to give plausible reasons for obtained differences in language tasks between socioeconomic groups. One might consider the most parsimonious interpretation of the data to be a difference in intelligence between the two groups of children. However, this would *not* seem to be the case with the present study. The reader will recall that both the standard subjects and the economically disadvantaged subjects were selected on the basis of having normal school achievement and/or intelligence test results as reported in the childrens' school records. No child in either group was included if he or she fell outside the normal limits on these tests.

It should be mentioned that one examiner administered the Token Test to all of the standard subjects and a different examiner gave it to all of the economically disadvantaged subjects. Perhaps some type of experimenter bias was operating. However, both examiners used the same scoring criteria. Furthermore, it seems unlikely that the obtained systematic differences in Token Test scores between the two groups would have occurred from uncontrolled variables in test administration. That is, how can one explain the observed results solely on the basis of differences in examiners?

In considering the results of this study, one must look at the test instrument itself. Is there something about the Token Test that inherently favors a middle-class population, or conversely penalizes an economically disadvantaged population? At least superficially, the items would seem to be relatively culture-fair. The tasks are all of the imperative construction, that is, they are all direct commands. Intuitively, both populations are presumed to be equally exposed to this grammatical structure. Furthermore, there would not appear to be any specific syntactical bias operating: The arrangement and interrelationships of words in the grammatical constructions of the sentences do not seem to favor the middle-class children. Or do they? Perhaps the linguistic style reflects what is sometimes referred to as *teacher's speech*. The commands, "Touch the little blue circle and the big white square" or "After I touch the green circle, you take the white square," appear to sound somewhat pedantic and stilted. Perhaps middle-class children are more responsive to this type of task, are able to attend to the instructions better, and thus achieve higher scores.

There is something else rather peculiar about the task itself. The whole test procedure is quite artificial. Certainly there is nothing exactly comparable in the real world to what is asked of the subject: some manipulations on command of plastic circles and squares. The children quickly realize that this is a strange test situation. It may well be that middle-class children are more test conscious than lower-class children, and are therefore more easily able to adapt or perform. Related to this issue, of course, is the matter of motivation. There is no doubt that subjects' motivation can influence Token Test results as with any test procedure. Perhaps, for some reason, economically disadvantaged children simply are less well motivated for this kind of a testing situation.

However, regardless of the basis for differences in scores between the two socioeconomic groups on the Token Test, it is clear that whenever the test is used to measure receptive language abilities among children, the examiner should be certain to use the appropriate normative data.

# APPENDIX

## PART I
Use only the large squares and the large circles.     (10 tokens)
1. Touch the red circle.
2. Touch the green square.
3. Touch the red square.
4. Touch the yellow circle.
5. Touch the blue circle.
6. Touch the green circle.
7. Touch the yellow square.
8. Touch the white circle.
9. Touch the blue square.
10. Touch the white square.

## PART II
Use the large and small squares and the large and small circles.     (20 tokens)
11. Touch the little yellow circle.
12. Touch the big green circle.
13. Touch the big yellow circle.
14. Touch the big blue square.
15. Touch the little green circle.
16. Touch the big red circle.
17. Touch the big white square.
18. Touch the little blue circle.
19. Touch the little green square.
20. Touch the big blue circle.

## PART III
Use only the large squares and the large circles.     (10 tokens)
21. Touch the yellow circle and the red square.
22. Touch the green square and the blue circle.
23. Touch the blue square and the yellow square.
24. Touch the white square and the red square.
25. Touch the white circle and the blue circle.
26. Touch the blue square and the white square.
27. Touch the blue square and the white circle.
28. Touch the green square and the blue circle.
29. Touch the red circle and the yellow square.
30. Touch the red square and the white circle.

## PART IV
Use the large and small squares and the large and small circles.     (20 tokens)
31. Touch the little yellow circle and the big green square.
32. Touch the little blue square and the little green circle.
33. Touch the big white square and the big red square.
34. Touch the big blue square and the big red square.
35. Touch the little blue square and the little yellow circle.
36. Touch the little blue circle and the little red circle.
37. Touch the big blue square and the big green square.
38. Touch the big blue circle and the big green circle.

39. *Touch the little red square and the little yellow circle.*
40. *Touch the little white square and the big red square.*

PART V

Use only the large squares and the large circles.    (10 tokens)

41. *Put the red circle on top of the green square.*
42. *Put the white square underneath the yellow circle.*
43. *Touch the blue circle with the red square.*
44. *Touch—with the blue circle—the red square.*
45. *Touch the blue circle and the red square.*
46. *Pick up the blue circle or the red square.*
47. *Put the green square away from the yellow square.*
48. *Put the white circle in front of the blue square.*
49. *If there is a black circle, pick up the red square.* (Note behavior.)
50. *Pick up the squares, except the yellow one.*
51. *Touch the white circle without using your right hand.*
52. *When I touch the green circle, you take the white square.* (Wait 5 sec before touching the green circle.)
53. *Put the green square beside the red circle.*
54. *Touch the squares slowly and the circles quickly.*
55. *Put the red circle between the yellow square and the green square.*
56. *Except for the green one, touch the circles.*
57. *Pick up the red circle—no, that's wrong!—the white square.*
58. *Instead of the white square, take the yellow circle.*
59. *Together with the yellow circle, take the blue circle.*
60. *After picking up the green square, touch the white circle.*
61. *Put the blue circle under the white square.*
62. *Before touching the yellow circle, pick up the red square.*

# V
## CEREBRAL LOCALIZATION OF TOKEN TEST PERFORMANCE

# 10

## Long-Term Stability of Hemispheric Scores on the Token Test Following Brain Bisection and Hemidecortication

ERAN ZAIDEL

De Renzi's and Vignolo's Token Test (1962) is a particularly suitable index of the lower limits of auditory language comprehension in the right cerebral hemisphere. This is partly due to the remarkable clinical usefulness and sensitivity of the test. It is very portable, simple to administer, and now commercially available from the Neuropsychology laboratory of the University of Victoria in British Columbia (Spreen & Benton, 1969). Moreover, it is a reliable measure of even subtle or latent aphasic disturbances, though it does not discriminate between clinical subtypes of aphasia (Orgass & Poeck, 1966; Poeck, Kerschensteiner, & Hartje, 1972). In particular, it is as good in diagnosing nonfluent aphasias due to anterior lesions of the dominant hemisphere as it is in diagnosing fluent aphasias following posterior left cerebral lesions. The fact that the test is poor in discriminating between the aphasic syndromes may seem paradoxical since the Token Test ostensibly measures the integrity of auditory language comprehension rather than speech. The explanation seems to be that the test is sensitive to disorders in short-term verbal memory which itself may depend on the integrity of motor speech programming (Zaidel, 1977). Thus short-term verbal memory is said to support a verbal rehearsal buffer which, in turn, is necessary for decoding long and context-free auditory messages. This explains in part why comprehension deficits are common in all forms of aphasia, including cases presenting predominantly motor disorders.

Another reason for the research interest in the Token Test is that it refers to a well circumscribed, miniature language system with a finite, simple universe of discourse. This system is easily amenable to experimental control yet is also rich enough to include a variety of linguistic, perceptual (mainly visuo-spatial), and cognitive operations. For example, the test combines linguistic aspects of reference in a completely unambiguous semantics and the more abstract grammatical structures of verbs, prepositions, conjunctions, and syntactic predication. The perceptual requirements of the test include shape, size, and color identification and discrimination and some memory, even though the demands on vision and manual control are simple enough to allow testing of mildly agnosic or apraxic neurological patients. In particular, since the test requires no verbal response and only very simple manual manipulations, it is suitable for separate unilateral administrations to the disconnected and isolated left and right hemispheres. Although the test involves a small universe of discourse, it is nonetheless natural in the sense that the linguistic, perceptual, and cognitive components are not logically matched or uniquely prespecified; alternative strategies for solving the instructions are possible, and error analysis reveals divergent patterns of breakdown.

In what follows I will discuss the long-term changes during a 3-5 year followup of laterality effects on the Token Test following cerebral commissurotomy and hemispherectomy. In commissurotomy (split brain) and hemispherectomy (hemidecortication) patients, the hemispheric differences in cognitive skills can be observed directly as differences of positive unilateral competence rather than being inferred from deficit. The results of initial testing were reported in Zaidel (1977). Here I will reassess the original laterality effects in the light of repeated testing and investigate the long- and short-term reliability of hemispheric scores on the test. There is virtually no published data on changes in Token Test scores as a function of recovery from aphasia. However, the sensitivity of the test to the presence of aphasia, together with its insensitivity to differential aphasic symptomatology suggest that improvement of Token Test scores will only be noticeable with radical spontaneous recovery in linguistic competence or with intervention training of skills specific to this test.

## METHODS AND PROCEDURE

### Subjects

The Token Test performances of four neurosurgical patients were sampled longitudinally, over periods of from 3 to 5 years. The case histories are summarized in Table 10.1. The two commissurotomy patients, N. G. and L. B., are part of the group operated on by Drs. P. J. Vogel and J. E. Bogen (Bogen & Vogel, 1975) and studied intensively in Dr. R. W. Sperry's laboratory at Caltech (Sperry, 1974). These two patients, a female and a male, were selected because they vary considerably in IQ, age at surgery, age when first symptoms occurred, and age when tested. They also present psychological evidence of less severe and less lateralized extracallosal damage than the other patients in this group. Thus, together, they are believed to better represent the range of the pure disconnection syndrome.

Patients R. S. and D. W., respectively, had dominant and nondominant hemispherectomy before puberty and for lesions incurred well after speech acquisition but before reading. R. S. was operated on by Drs. Vogel and Bogen. She had progressively worsening aphasia prior to left hemispherectomy and afterwards presented a generally stable and unique aphasic syndrome characterized by nonfluent speech, a strong semantic focus, partly remissed anomia, and by skillful singing, good intonation, and frequent nonverbal imitation. Her auditory comprehension surpassed her speech and she had no functional reading or writing. R. S. has since died at age 16 from recurrence of the tumor. D. W. is a patient of Dr. I. G. Gill and was operated on by Dr. E. Green. His comprehension and speech are relatively intact but he has chronic dyslexia of the dyseidetic type (Boder, 1971), as well as dysgraphia and dyscalculia. These are accompanied by severe visuo-spatial and constructive deficits.

*Procedure*

Patients R. S. and D. W. were tested in the standard manner in free-vision, with no special apparatus. Patients N. G. and L. B. were fitted with individual scleral contact lenses on their dominant, right eye for ocular scanning with one hemisphere at a time (Zaidel, 1975a). This technique permits continuous lateralization of complex visual stimuli together with visual monitoring and guidance of manual control (see Figure 10.1).

The Token Test was explained and demonstrated verbally and visually in free-vision without the lens system. The test was then administered in the left visual half-field (LVF) with left hand responses and, a week later, in the RVF with right hand responses. In this way the positive competence of one hemisphere was compared directly with that of its sister hemisphere with which it is automatically matched for sex, age, education, etc. The test was also administered, yet another week later, in free-field. The commissurotomy patients were tested again five years

**TABLE 10.1**
*Summary of Case Histories*

| Patient | Sex | Reason for surgery | Surgery | Age at surgery | Years postop at testing (1975) | Age at onset of symptoms | IQ history[a] Preop | IQ history[a] Postop | Predominant extracallosal damage |
|---|---|---|---|---|---|---|---|---|---|
| N.G. | F | Intractable epilepsy | Complete cerebral commissurotomy: Single stage midline section of anterior commissures, corpus callosum (and presumably psalterium), massa intermedia and right fornix. Surgical approach by retraction of the right hemisphere. | 30 | 12 | 18 | Wechsler-Bellvue 76 (79, 74) at age 30 | WAIS 77 (83, 71) at age 35 | RH(BI) |
| L.B. | M | Intractable epilepsy | As above but massa intermedia was not visualized. | 13 | 10 | 3:6 | WISC 113 (119, 108) at age 13 | WAIS 106 (110, 100) at age 16 | RH |
| R.S. | F | Glioma | Left (dominant) hemispherectomy including caudate nucleus and upper portion of thalamus. Partial tumor removal via a left parietal incision at age 8. Occipito-parietal lesion for installment and revision of a ventro-jugular shunt. Died at age 16:10 of recurrence of tumor. | 10 | 6 | 8 | Kuhlman-Anderson 100 at age 8 | WISC 56 (63, 55) at age 13 | — |
| D.W. | M | Intractable epilepsy | Right hemispherectomy presumably sparing basal ganglia and thalamus. Frontal topectomy at age 6:11. Left-handed prior to hemispherectomy but RH amytal showed speech lateralization to LH. | 7:9 | 12 | 6:7 | Stanford-Binet 125 at age 3:6 | WISC 67 (80, 60) at age 16:6 | — |

[a] IQ is expressed, full scale IQ (verbal IQ, performance IQ).

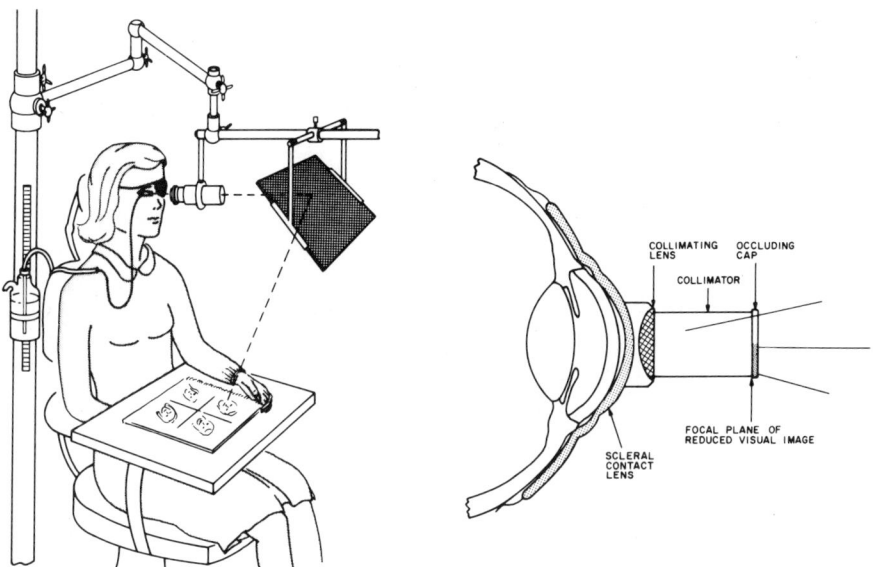

**FIGURE 10.1.** *The experimental setup (left) and contact lens assembly (right) used for ocular scanning by one visual half-field at a time.*

later. In this case the right and left hemispheres were tested on the same day. Patient R. S. was tested three times in the course of 3 years and patient D. W. was tested three times in the course of 4 years. The scores of these two patients were compared with each other.

The Token Test instructions were read aloud to the subject by the examiner in the usual manner while the display was restricted to one visual half-field. Thus both hemispheres could hear the instruction but only the "seeing hemisphere" could respond correctly. The tokens in the array were placed randomly and scrambled after each instruction in order to prevent cues about the position of the tokens in the left visual half field from reaching the left hemisphere (LH) during RH performance through possible ipsilateral manual (left hand) or visual (LVF) feedback. The initial testing (Zaidel, 1977) showed that it was not necessary to paint the tokens on identical plaques in order to eliminate ipsilateral somesthetic cues of shape and size during unilateral presentations; similar laterality effects were observed on De Renzi and Vignolo's version of the test (1962) administered with physically identical plaques, and on Spreen and Benton's version of the test (1969) administered with the standard plastic tokens.

In retesting, I used Spreen and Benton's test with slight modifications. The first change, already mentioned, was that the chips were randomized rather than arranged in a standard order of rows of uniform size and shape. The second change consisted of small differences in scoring conventions for partial credit (see Appendix).

Both pass–fail (Boller & Vignolo, 1966) and weighted scores (Orgass & Poeck, 1966) were computed. In the pass–fail scoring system each instruction is worth one point which is awarded only if the instruction is executed faultlessly. Weighted-scoring, on the other hand, awards partial credit for the relevant parts of the message which were executed correctly. Weighted scores are necessarily somewhat arbitrary since the original intent of the subject cannot be verified. Here, a principle of lenient scoring was adopted and order was not enforced. Although some verb errors did occur in the execution of the last part of the test by the disconnected RHs, the possibility cannot be ruled out that more RH errors would have occurred were it not for some help by the LHs through ipsilateral motor control. The modified test and its scoring conventions are presented in the Appendix.

## RESULTS AND DISCUSSION

The longitudinal data are summarized in Table 10.2. Unilateral raw scores on each part of the test are given for all patients. Total pass–fail and weighted scores are shown as well.

### Laterality Effects

The unilateral pass–fail scores of each patient are compared in Figure 10.2, and the mean left and right hemisphere patterns of performance on subsequent parts of the test are shown in Figure 10.3. These data include the original administration of the test (Zaidel, 1977) as well as the more recent followup testing. It is clear that the LHs made few errors and are within the upper 25% range of normal adults. The RHs, on the other hand, suffered a severe deficit, comparable to that of heterogeneous aphasics. This difference between matched left and right hemispheres is highly significant statistically. There was no significant difference between the scores of the disconnected LHs and the respective patients' scores in free-vision. It follows that the LH controls performance on this test when administered in the standard manner. The last part of the test alone discriminated reliably between the two hemispheres just as it does between aphasic and nonaphasic brain-damaged patients (Spellacy & Spreen, 1969). In Figures 10.2, 10.3, and 10.4, the unilateral scores are compared with the percentile ranks of left brain-

**TABLE 10.2**
*Left and Right Hemisphere Scores on Spreen and Benton's Token Test[a]*

| Patient | Hemisphere | Date of testing | Part A | | Part B | | Part C | | Part D | | Part E | | Part F | | Total number correct | | Total percent correct | |
|---|---|---|---|---|---|---|---|---|---|---|---|---|---|---|---|---|---|---|
| | | | PF | WS | PF | WS | PF | WS | PF | WS | PF | WS | PF | WS | PF | WS | PF | WS |
| Maximum score[b] | | | 7 | 7 | 4 | 8 | 4 | 12 | 4 | 16 | 4 | 24 | 16 | 94 | 39 | 159 | 100 | 100 |
| N.G. | RH | 2/7/73 | 7 | 7 | 4 | 8 | 1 | 7 | 1 | 11 | 0 | 18 | 4 | 63 | 17 | 114 | 44 | 72 |
| | | 3/1/78 | 6 | 6 | 2 | 5 | 4 | 9 | 0 | 8 | 0 | 12 | 3 | 68 | 15 | 108 | 38 | 68 |
| | LH | 2/20/73 | 7 | 7 | 4 | 8 | 2 | 10 | 4 | 16 | 3 | 23 | 13 | 86 | 33 | 150 | 85 | 94 |
| | | 3/1/78 | 7 | 7 | 4 | 8 | 4 | 12 | 4 | 16 | 4 | 24 | 15 | 92 | 38 | 159 | 97 | 100 |
| | BI | 3/3/78 | 7 | 7 | 4 | 8 | 4 | 12 | 4 | 16 | 4 | 24 | 15 | 91 | 39 | 158 | 100 | 99 |
| L.B. | RH | 2/5/73 | 5 | 5 | 3 | 7 | 3 | 11 | 0 | 9 | 1 | 20 | 6 | 74 | 18 | 126 | 46 | 79 |
| | | 3/1/78 | 6 | 6 | 3 | 7 | 2 | 10 | 0 | 8 | 2 | 21 | 6 | 69 | 19 | 121 | 49 | 76 |
| | LH | 2/7/73 | 7 | 7 | 4 | 8 | 4 | 12 | 4 | 16 | 4 | 24 | 14 | 89 | 37 | 156 | 95 | 98 |
| | | 3/1/78 | 7 | 7 | 4 | 8 | 4 | 12 | 4 | 16 | 4 | 24 | 16 | 92 | 39 | 159 | 100 | 100 |
| | BI | 3/3/73 | 7 | 7 | 4 | 8 | 4 | 12 | 4 | 16 | 4 | 24 | 14 | 90 | 37 | 157 | 95 | 99 |
| R.S. | RH | 3/1/73 | 5 | 5 | 2 | 6 | 2 | 10 | 0 | 8 | 0 | 12 | 0 | 44 | 9 | 85 | 8 | 53 |
| | | 5/21/75 | 6 | 6 | 1 | 5 | 2 | 10 | 0 | 8 | 0 | 14 | 0 | 55 | 9 | 98 | 8 | 62 |
| | | 4/28/76 | 5 | 5 | 1 | 3 | 0 | 6 | 0 | 7 | 0 | 14 | 0 | 49 | 6 | 84 | 15 | 53 |
| D.W. | LH | 3/3/73 | 7 | 7 | 4 | 8 | 4 | 12 | 4 | 16 | 1 | 21 | 13 | 86 | 33 | 150 | 85 | 94 |
| | | 7/16/73 | 7 | 7 | 4 | 8 | 4 | 12 | 4 | 16 | 3 | 22 | 15 | 91 | 37 | 156 | 95 | 98 |
| | | 2/3/77 | 7 | 7 | 4 | 8 | 4 | 12 | 4 | 16 | 4 | 24 | 15 | 91 | 38 | 158 | 97 | 99 |

[a] PF = pass-fail score; WS = weighted score (partial credit); LH = left hemisphere; BI = bilateral or free-vision score.
[b] The Appendix shows a revised version.

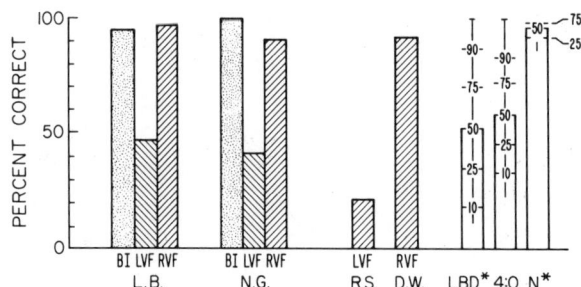

**FIGURE 10.2.** *Unilateral pass–fail scores on Spreen and Benton's Token Test (1969). Mean longitudinal data. Percentile ranks of left brain-damaged patients (LBD) (McClellan et al., 1973), of four-year-old children (Zaidel, 1977) and of normal control subjects (N) (McClellan et al., 1973) are shown for comparison. BI = bilateral score, in free-field testing, LVF = left visual half-field testing (right hemisphere), RVF = right visual half-field testing (left hemisphere), an asterisk indicates data obtained with De Renzi and Vignolo's version of the test using a fixed display.*

damaged patients, 4-year-old children, and normal controls on identical or similar versions of the Token Test.

Control tests established that both hemispheres could match tokens by color, shape, and size. The disconnected RHs could also understand the color and size adjectives, and color nouns when they occurred in isolation, but, as Figure 10.3 illustrates, they deteriorated progressively as the test instructions got longer. For both weighted and pass–fail scores, the (LH − RH) differences are statistically significant and the (LH − free-field) disparities are not. But the weighted scores of the RHs are higher than their pass–fail scores when both measures are expressed as age scores or percentile ranks relative to aphasics. This means that the RHs were selectively impaired in their ability to retain the whole message in the correct order, or equivalently, that they were relatively adept in

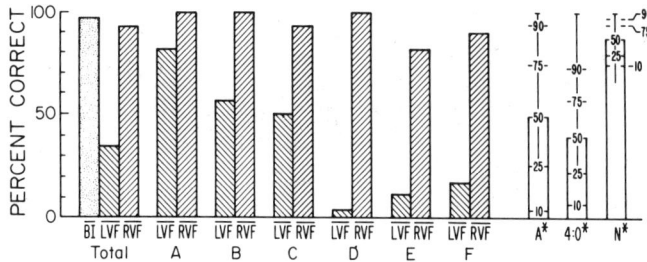

**FIGURE 10.3.** *Mean unilateral pass–fail scores on Spreen and Benton's Token Test. The longitudinal data is compared with the percentile ranks of left brain-damaged patients, 4-year-old children, and normal controls (see Figure 10.2).*

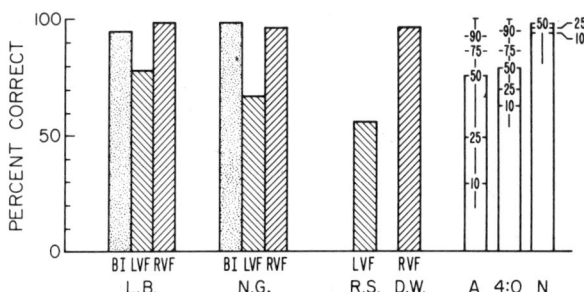

**FIGURE 10.4.** *Unilateral weighted scores on Spreen and Benton's Token Test. Longitudinal data. Percentile ranks of aphasics (A) and of normal controls (N) (both from Spreen and Benton, 1969) as well as of 4-year-old children (Zaidel, 1977) are shown for comparison.*

retrieving part of the instruction even when they did not get it all. (See Figure 10.4.)

The data in Figures 10.2–10.5 are not coextensive with those reported in Zaidel (1977). Here, the data with De Renzi and Vignolo's version are omitted but included is all the information obtained in the several years followup with the Spreen and Benton version. For this larger data base, the pattern of pass-fail scores on subsequent parts of the test again shows a bigger deficit for the RHs on Parts D and E than on Part F of the test. Part F, which is more difficult for aphasics, is more complex linguistically but Parts D and E have a higher load on memory. Independent evidence exists (Zaidel, 1978b) that the RH is selectively more sensitive to extralinguistic parameters of the message, such as word difficulty (indexed by frequency or by age of acquisition) and especially memory load, than to linguistic constraints such as grammatical structure (e.g., syntactic transformational derivational complexity). Indeed,

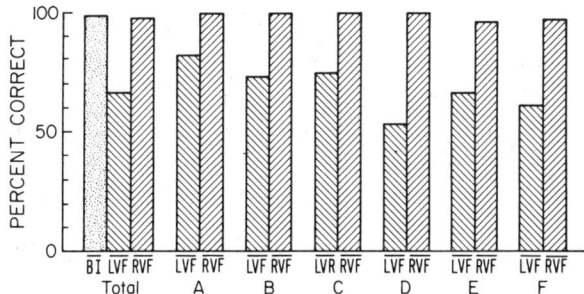

**FIGURE 10.5.** *Mean unilateral weighted scores on the whole Token Test and on its parts. Longitudinal data.*

**TABLE 10.3**
*Error Analysis*

| | | Parts A–E Reference | | | Part F Reference | | | | |
|---|---|---|---|---|---|---|---|---|---|
| | | Size | Color | Shape | Shape | Color | Verbs | Spatial prepositions | Particles |
| *Number* of errors by category for each hemisphere[a] | | | | | | | | | |
| Maximum number | | 12 | 29 | 26 | 28 | 26 | 16 | 7 | 15 |
| N.G. | | | | | | | | | |
| RH | 2/7/73 | 8 | 6 | 2 | 12 | 4 | 2 | 1 | 8 |
| | 3/1/78 | 10 | 14 | 3 | 8 | 7 | 1 | 3 | 3 |
| LH | 2/20/73 | 1 | 0 | 2 | 1 | 0 | 0 | 0 | 4 |
| | 3/1/78 | 0 | 0 | 0 | 0 | 0 | 0 | 0 | 0 |
| BI | 3/3/73 | 0 | 0 | 0 | 0 | 1 | 0 | 0 | 0 |
| L.B. | | | | | | | | | |
| RH | 2/5/73 | 6 | 9 | 0 | 8 | 7 | 0 | 0 | 1 |
| | 3/1/78 | 8 | 7 | 0 | 7 | 10 | 1 | 0 | 1 |

|  |  | 1 | 2 | 3 | 4 | 5 | 6 | 7 | 8 |
|---|---|---|---|---|---|---|---|---|---|
| LH | 2/7/73 | 0 | 0 | 0 | 1 | 2 | 0 | 0 | 0 |
|  | 3/1/78 | 0 | 0 | 0 | 0 | 0 | 0 | 0 | 0 |
| BI | 3/3/73 | 0 | 0 | 0 | 1 | 0 | 0 | 0 | 1 |
| R.S. |  |  |  |  |  |  |  |  |  |
| RH | 3/1/73 | 7 | 16 | 3 | 11 | 21 | 3 | 1 | 9 |
|  | 5/21/75 | 9 | 15 | 0 | 6 | 19 | 4 | 1 | 4 |
|  | 4/28/76 | 10 | 17 | 4 | 12 | 21 | 0 | 1 | 5 |
| D.W. |  |  |  |  |  |  |  |  |  |
| LH | 3/3/73 | 0 | 1 | 2 | 0 | 6 | 0 | 0 | 0 |
|  | 7/16/73 | 0 | 0 | 0 | 1 | 0 | 0 | 0 | 0 |
|  | 2/3/77 | 0 | 0 | 0 | 0 | 1 | 0 | 0 | 0 |

Summary of *percent* of RH errors by category

|  | 1 | 2 | 3 | 4 | 5 | 6 | 7 | 8 |
|---|---|---|---|---|---|---|---|---|
| N.G. and L.B. | 67 | 31 | 4 | 31 | 27 | 6 | 14 | 22 |
| R.S. | 72 | 55 | 9 | 35 | 65 | 15 | 14 | 40 |
| RH mean | 69 | 39 | 6 | 32 | 40 | 9 | 14 | 28 |

|  | Color (Parts A-E) | Shape (Parts A-E) |
|---|---|---|
| RH mean | 40 | 20 |

[a] The Appendix shows a revised version.

there is a nonsignificant Spearman rank order correlation coefficient between item difficulty for aphasics and for the RHs on the last part of the test (Zaidel, 1977). Similarly, whereas the incidence of particle errors in the last part of the test (Table 10.3) is comparable for the RHs (24%) and for aphasics (26%, estimated from De Renzi and Vignolo, 1962), the RHs had many more reference errors (36% as against 7%). Nevertheless, our data are consistent with the view that the RH can serve as a basis for partial language recovery from aphasia following left or dominant hemisphere lesions. Indeed, on the average the RH of patient N. G. ranked around the 36th percentile relative to 208 heterogeneous aphasics, L. B.'s RH ranked approximately in the 53rd percentile and R. S. ranked about the 33rd percentile (see Figure 10.4).

We may summarize the observed laterality effects by noting that the LH seems highly specialized for decoding Token Test instructions. There is no evidence from our data for a RH contribution to the task (cf. Swisher & Sarno, 1969), which would result in a mild unilateral LH deficit, even though the administration maximized the need for visuospatial cues because of the random display. Rather, the Token Test seems to delineate the lower limits of auditory language comprehension in the RH. RH comprehension fails when the sentence is long, contains ordered information and is nonredundant. This RH deficit may be attributable to a severely limited short term verbal memory which is necessary for verbal rehearsal and which may, in turn, be due to the absence of speech and phonetic analyzers in this hemisphere (Zaidel, 1977, 1978b).

*Long-Term Changes in Token Test Scores*

Figures 10.6–10.9 illustrate the long-term stability of unilateral Token Test scores, both in terms of the pass–fail (see Figures 10.6 and 10.7) and of the weighted (see Figures 10.8 and 10.9) measures. This long-term stability applies both to scores on the whole test (see Figures 10.6 and 10.8) as well as to the difference in scores between Parts D–E (which are mnestically loaded) and Part F (linguistically complex) (see Figures 10.7 and 10.9). Clearly, overall scores on the test, especially for the right hemispheres, remain stable. There is a slight trend for weighted scores to decrease with time in the RHs and to increase with time in the LHs but this trend is not significant. The pattern of a fixed RH deficit contrasts with three other patterns of long-term change in unilateral performances on different psycholinguistic tasks by the same patients.

The first strikingly different pattern involves improvement in the auditory vocabulary of the RH. Patient R. S. with a dominant hemi-

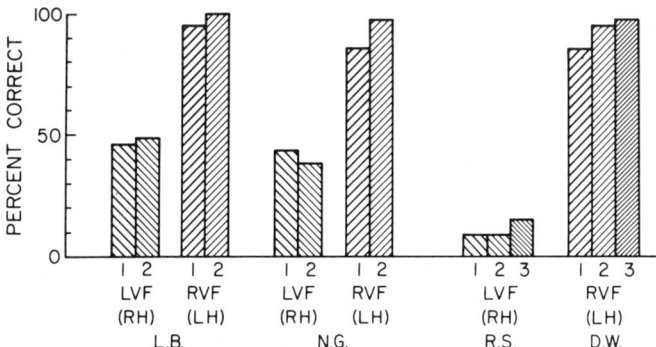

**FIGURE 10.6.** *Long-term changes in the pass–fail Token Test scores of each hemisphere. 1 = original testing; 2,3 = subsequent retestings (see Table 10.2).*

spherectomy illustrates this pattern best. During the same 3-year period when her Token Test scores remained virtually unchanged, her auditory vocabulary improved at a rate equivalent to that of a normal child with the same mental age. In other words, she increased from an equivalent psycholinguistic age of 13:3 to that of 16:7 on the Peabody Picure Vocabulary Test (Dunn, 1965) used as a measure of receptive vocabulary (Zaidel, 1976b). R. S.'s auditory vocabulary scores were also much more sensitive to changes in her neurological status, especially in the form of a progressive deficit with increasing hydrocephalus due to malfunction of a ventrojugular shunt and occasionally dramatic improvements following shunt revision (Bogen, Kumar, Johnson, Ozgur, Smith, Thale, Wit-

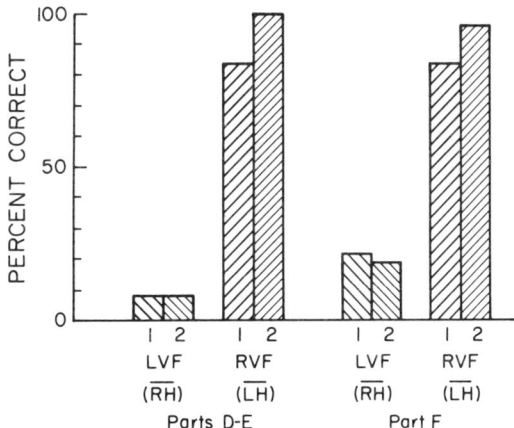

**FIGURE 10.7.** *Long-term changes in unilateral pass–fail scores on parts D–E versus part F of the Token Test.*

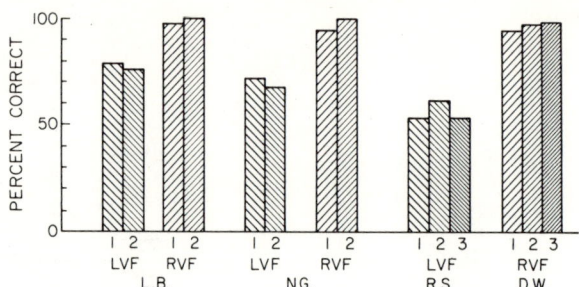

**FIGURE 10.8.** *Long-term changes in unilateral weighted Token Test scores.*

ton, & Zaidel, 1978). Table 10.4 shows the long-term changes in R. S.'s PPVT scores during a period of 5 years.

We should perhaps not expect a comparable growth of auditory vocabulary in the adult disconnected RHs to that found in the young hemispherectomy patient. But case R. S. is important because it demonstrates that the observed upper (Peabody) and lower (Token Test) limits of linguistic performance in the RH are both points in a continuous and progressive developmental process rather than the consequences of sudden reorganization due to surgery or trauma, such as regression to a lower level or loss of a skill. Thus, auditory vocabulary is highly developed naturally in the RH; the RHs of patients L.B., N.G. and R.S. reached mental ages of 16:3, 11:0, and 11:9, respectively (Zaidel, 1976a), on the Peabody test. Furthermore, the meaning that the RH associates with lexical items though rich, seems connotative and diffuse in contrast to lexical semantics in the LH which seems to be more denotative and

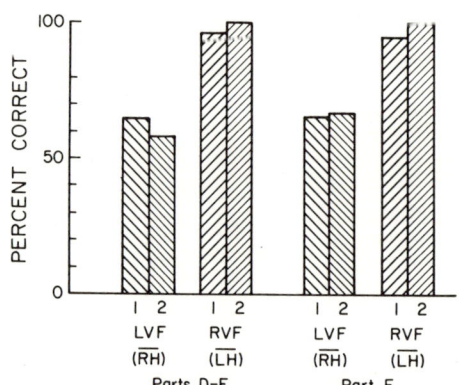

**FIGURE 10.9.** *Long-term changes in unilateral weighted scores on parts D–E versus part F of the Token Test.*

**TABLE 10.4**
*Record of Longitudinal Testing of Auditory Vocabulary in Patient R.S. with the Peabody Picture Vocabulary Test*

| Examiner | Testing date | Age | Raw score | Verbal IQ | Mental age |
|---|---|---|---|---|---|
| Karol Fishler | 11/ 8/71 | 12:2 | 60 | 64 | 6:10 |
| Peggy Gott | 6/12/72 | 12:9 | 64 | 66 | 7:8 |
| Eran Zaidel | 12/19/72 | 13:3 | 66 | 68 | 8:1 |
| Eran Zaidel | 3/17/74 | 14:6 | 67 | 67 | 8:3 |
| Eran Zaidel | 4/21/76 | 16:7 | 84 | 78 | 11:9 |

precise. Also, RH perception of spoken and printed words seems to be by Gestalt pattern matching rather than by feature analysis (Zaidel, 1978b). It is plausible, therefore, that auditory and, to a somewhat lesser extent, visual lexical semantics calls for bilateral cooperation in the normal brain.

On the other hand, the Token Test identifies the inherent limitation in the RH ability to retrieve meaning from sequences of lexical items even when each word can be understood in isolation. I have shown here that this inability to decode phrases with context-free, ordered, multiple references seems to characterize RH style quite early and shows no evidense of compensatory readjustment thereafter. There is a weaker long-term stability in the grammatical ability of the disconnected and isolated RHs. Indeed, the long-term change in error pattern of the RHs for different categories of words in the Token Test (see Figure 10.10) shows that the RHs tend to have an increasing difficulty in retrieving the reference or content words from the adjectival modifying phrases of the Token Test instructions; they have an overall diminishing deficit, on the other hand, in interpreting verbs and particles, which are linguistically more marked and perceptually more prominent in the sentences.

To say that the adult RH remains at the 4-year-old level on the Token Test is not necessarily to imply that the two hemispheres develop equipotentially for language until age 4 or so, at which point the LH is said to further specialize in linguistic performance whereas the RH remains forever arrested at that stage of linguistic ability (Zaidel, 1978a). This is apparently not so because the RH does not represent any recognizable stage in first language acquisition: It has no speech, has a rich auditory lexicon, a substantial though smaller reading vocabulary, and very poor reading and comprehension of long phrases. In fact, even when a given RH reaches some age level, that is, in a sense the same linguistic competence, as a child of a certain age, it still exhibits distinctly

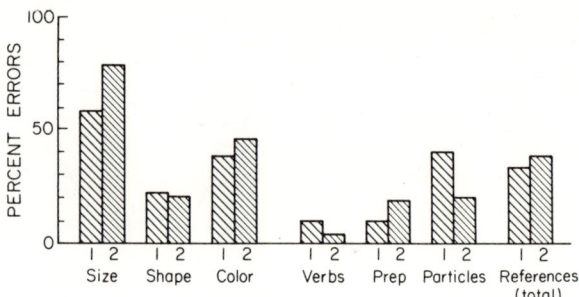

**FIGURE 10.10.** *Long-term changes in mean error scores of the right hemispheres.*

different performance patterns revealed by different kinds of errors. This is true for the Token Test (Zaidel, 1977) and it can also be shown for other better developed linguistic structures in the RH (Zaidel, 1978a).

The second pattern that contrasts with the stable and chronic RH deficit on the Token Test occurs in the long-term changes of the mental age profiles of patients R. S. and D. W. with dominant and nondominant hemispherectomy, respectively, on the Illinois Test of Psycholinguistic Abilities (ITPA) (Zaidel, in press). Each patient showed a selective long-term improvement on a few subtests of the ITPA (Kirk, McCarthy, & Kirk, 1969) and a selective deterioration on a few others. But the subtests showing these changes are not the same in both patients. Thus, a three-year followup of patient D. W. revealed gains in auditory closure, manual expression, visual reception and grammatic closure, and losses in verbal expression and visual sequential memory (Zaidel, in press). R. S., on the other hand, suffered her biggest losses in visual reception and manual expression, both tests in which D. W. gained during the same period. Her main gains were in visual association and visual closure (Zaidel, in press). Such gains may be due to either spontaneous development of original hemispheric skills, or they may signal functional reorganization, perhaps at the expense of innate skills. Long-term deterioration, on the other hand, seems to invariably signal loss due to readjustment. The relevant point here is that the skills indexed by the Token Test must be so fundamentally limited in the RH that they do not allow compensatory redevelopment.

The third pattern of unilateral long-term change occurs in the ITPA profiles of six commissurotomy patients in free-field. Free-field performance presumably expresses LH control and competence. Both profiles show, first, subnormal scores which seem to reflect substantial

LH deficits on most of these tests, in sharp contrast with the symptom-free clinical impression. Second; there is a large variability across subtests and patients so that none of the six patients presented a profile which is equivalent to a normal child at the same age level. However, comparison of the free-field ITPA profiles of individual patients in 1972 and 1975 reveals a general tendency towards improved performance as well as a regression towards the mean scores of a normal child with the same composite (overall) psycholinguistic age. In other words, there is an apparent trend toward more normal scores and reduced variability.

*Short-Term Variability in RH Token Test Scores*

Although total pass–fail as well as weighted Token Test scores in the RHs remain constantly low, there is evidence that the RH is inherently more variable in its "local" performance on specific items than is the LH. This variability occurs also in the short-term and is demonstrated by a relative inconsistency of error patterns on individual Token Test instructions. In order to compare the degree of association between all subsequent administrations of the Token Test to the same left and right hemispheres, I have computed Kendall's coefficient of concordance, $W$, for ranking of weighted score in each administration (Siegel, 1956). The results are shown in Table 10.5. In all cases, the LHs showed a higher uniformity or concordance than the corresponding RHs.

I have also compared the variability of test–retest pass–fail scores in the two hemispheres by dividing the Token Test instructions into three

**TABLE 10.5**
*Kendall's Coefficient of Concordance W for All Subsequent Administrations of the Token Test to Each Hemisphere*[a]

| Hemisphere | Measure | Patient | | |
| --- | --- | --- | --- | --- |
| | | L.B. | N.G. | D.W. vs R.S. |
| LH | $W$[b] | .9755 | .9796 | .8507 |
| | $\chi^2$ | 68.7308** | 69.9746** | 91.5464*** |
| RH | $W$ | .9499 | .8947 | .7797 |
| | $\chi^2$ | 70.2424** | 65.507* | 83.796*** |

[a]Ranking of weighted scores used correction for ties.
[b]$W$ takes values between 0 and +1 with higher values signifying higher association or agreement. For large $N$, $\chi^2 = K(N-1)W$ so that the significance level of $W$ may be obtained from a $\chi^2$ table with $df = N - 1$.
*$p < .01$.
**$p < .005$.
***$p < .001$.

categories for each hemisphere: those that yielded the same unilateral scores on test–retest, those that yielded higher scores on retest, and those that yielded lower scores on retest. I then intended to perform the nonparametric $\chi^2$ test for two independent samples on the resulting frequency data in order to determine whether the test–retest difference was greater in one hemisphere than in the other. Because some expected frequencies were too small, I had to collapse the data into two categories: (a) number of items with the same score in test and retest, and (b) number of items with different scores between test and retest. The results of the analysis are shown in Table 10.6. Even though the statistical test does not use much of the data, significant differences were obtained between the test–retest agreement in the LH and that in the RH of both patients N.G. and L.B. The RHs had a consistently higher incidence of items with different scores in test and retest.

Actually, the above demonstrations of greater RH than LH variability in performance on individual test instructions are not conclusive. The smaller LH variability may, in fact, be due to its higher level of performance. Strictly speaking, the variability of the two hemispheres needs to be compared on tests of equal difficulty for both. Such was approximately the case for Raven's Colored Progressive Matrices Test (Zaidel, Zaidel, & Sperry, 1978). There, the RHs were more variable than the corresponding LHs, though equally as competent. An alternative procedure to comparing the variability of the two hemispheres with each other is to compare each to the normal range of variability in a group of appropriate control subjects, such as normal children, with the same respective performance level. But such data are not available for the Token Test so that the comparison cannot be undertaken at the present time.

I have observed a similar pattern of highly variable RH performance in subsequent administrations of many tasks, even when the intertest interval was quite short (Zaidel, 1973). This unique characteris-

**TABLE 10.6**
*The $\chi^2$ Test for Two Independent Samples Comparing the Difference between Pass–Fail Test–Retest Scores in the LH with Those in the RH*[a]

|  | N.G. | L.B. | D.W. versus R.S. |
|---|---|---|---|
| $\chi^2$ | 4.81* | 8.74** | .1 |

[a] A correction for continuity was used.
*$p < .05$.
**$p < .005$.

tic of information processing in the RH may be related to its selectively poor error-correction ability, which in turn may be attributed to the fact that the RH solves problems nonalgorithmically, that is, without an internal step-by-step model of its own solution process which can be interrogated and updated (Zaidel, 1978c). It is interesting that this presumed inherent instability in RH problem solving ability remains local and does not seem to affect the total performance level. Similar patterns are commonly observed in learning experiments with animals and in the short-term lability of the cognitive competence of brain-damaged patients. Thus, monkeys are said to have mastered a problem when they reach criteria of about 90% correct responses because they rarely perform at 100%, even when they have clearly learned to the task. When assessing patients with cognitive deficit due to focal cortical lesions, a major problem is to decide whether the task is to document constant and reliable levels of performance or optimal even if only occasional competence. In the case of the RH, we can model the variability statistically, and we may hypothesize that the cause is some attentional shifts. But the mechanism remains to be determined.

## CONCLUSIONS

This pattern of local variability but global stability in the RH style of information processing may have some consequences to hemispheric differences in learning rates and optimal instructional strategies for each. For instance, our data (Zaidel, 1978c) suggest that the RH should not be taught by feedback during trial-and-error, nor is it likely to learn a concept from exposure to one example of it (Zaidel, 1978b). These methods are more effective for LH learning. For the RH, multiple, redundant, complete, and concrete models of the solution process are apparently more appropriate.

### Prospects

The foregoing discussion has important implications for the use of the Token Test as a measure of recovery from aphasia. We have shown that the requisite abilities are highly specialized in the LH and that the RH shows some "local" short-term lability, that is, that its performance on specific instructions is not always predictable. But the RH has stable global Token Test scores both in the short- and long-terms. The short-term variability requires caution in interpreting the reliability though not the validity of the Token Test, at least where error analysis is concerned. It follows that when properly repeated, the Token Test is uniquely suitable for detecting pure LH recovery in aphasia. Such recovery is likely to take place in the LH. The possibility that recovery signals RH assumption of certain linguistic skills previously represented in the LH and now shifting to the RH at the expense of traditional RH functions, cannot be ruled out and deserves further study.

It is a fundamental and still unresolved issue in rehabilitation theory whether recovery from cognitive deficit following circumscribed cerebral damage is due to progressive restoration of function to the damaged tissue which resumes its original roles, or whether, on the contrary, functional recovery signals compensatory adjustment of residual brain structures to the new task. In the case of acquired language deficit, these alternatives prescribe different approaches to therapy. If the goal is to retrain the damaged LH skills, then it makes sense to improve the patient's ability to perform Token Test instructions per se (Holland & Sonderman, 1974) using various strategies such as delayed response (Liles & Brookshire, 1975). If, on the other hand, the goal is to effect RH takeover of some comprehension skills then the data presented in this chapter suggest that "Token Test Therapy" will be ineffectual. Rather, semantic and pragmatic aspects of the communication context should be emphasized and their redundancy exploited.

It remains to be determined whether specialized training can improve Token Test performance in the RH. In particular, it was found that aphasic's comprehension of Token Test commands can be improved by inserting 2–5 sec pauses into the instructions (Liles & Brookshire, 1975; Salvatore, 1975), or by imposing a 5–10 sec delay before allowing the aphasic to respond (Yorkston, Marshall, & Butler, 1977). Holland and Whitney (this volume) also suggested that a similar facilitation can occur when the rate of presentation of Token Test instructions is slowed down. If similar manipulations fail to improve the performance of the disconnected and isolated RH on the Token Test then it follows that the aphasic's improvement is due to readjustment in the LH mechanisms alone.

Another interesting question concerns the effect of language modality on Token Test performance by aphasic patients. Will a reading version of the Token Test be performed better or worse than the auditory version by an aphasic who is not severely alexic? Results with the disconnected RHs (Zaidel, 1978b) suggest that they will not benefit from the continuous presence of the printed instructions. It seems that the linguistic message needs to be stored in some intermediate internal representation before it can be properly decoded. This intermediate representation is the same for visual and auditory information and the mechanism underlying it, perhaps phonetically supported short-term verbal memory, is nonfunctional in the RH. If, indeed, the RH turns out to gain no advantage with a reading version of the Token Test whereas certain aphasics do, then this will be further evidence that the damaged LH rather than the intact RH supports the comprehension process in these aphasics.

## ACKNOWLEDGMENTS

Thanks to Dahlia Zaidel and Charles R. Hamilton for useful comments on the manuscript. Mary-Beth Köppel, Carole E. Johnson, and Leslie L. Wolcott have assisted in different stages of this work. Financial support was provided by NIMH awards GM-57881 and Career Scientist Development Award MH-00179 as well as by Biomedical Research Support Program grant No. RR07003 to the author, and by USPHS grant MH-03372 and NSF grant BMS-76-01629 to R. W. Sperry.

## APPENDIX

## SCORING CONVENTIONS FOR THE TOKEN TEST[a]

A. *General*

1. Two methods of scoring are used, (*a*) pass–fail, and (*b*) weighted scores. In pass–fail scoring, each instruction is worth one point which is awarded only if no relevant error occurs. Maximum pass–fail score is 39 (in the short version 16, see A.4). Weighted scoring, on the other hand, awards partial credit for the relevant parts of the message which were executed correctly. In the test form each scorable item of each instruction is underlined and is worth one point. For example, if the subject touches the large yellow circle in response to "touch the *large green circle*," then he is credited with two out of three possible points. A principle of lenient weighted scoring is adopted and order is not enforced. For example, if in response to "touch the *large white square* and the *small yellow circle*," the subject touches the large yellow circle and the small red square, then he is credited with 3 rather than 2 out of 6 possible points. In Part F of the test, the principle of lenient scoring applies to all parts of the instruction. For example, if assuming an error on the verb maximizes the score on the reference and thus on the whole instruction, then this is the adopted interpretation. It should be noted that weighted scoring is somewhat arbitrary since the original intent of the subject is often unknown. The maximum weighted score is 163 (in the short version 80, see A.4).

2. Except in Parts A and B, instructions should not be repeated until the subject has responded, even if he has to resort to guessing. If there is an error, his answer is recorded, and the examiner should say, "Let's try this again," and repeat the instruction. The subject's second response is then recorded and scored separately only for research purposes.

3. The tokens should be placed randomly and the manipulated ones should be scrambled after each response to prevent perseverations and memory cues. For research

[a] Based on Test 11 in Spreen and Benton's Neurosensory Center Comprehensive Examination for Aphasia, University of Victoria, 1969.

and comparison purposes, an unscrambled version of the test can also be used with the following fixed layout:

R B Y W G
B R W G Y
W B Y R G
Y G R B W

This unscrambled version is the standard administration in Spreen and Benton's version of the Token Test (1969).

4. A shorter version of the test consists of the 16 instructions marked with an asterisk (*). This version gives a maximum pass-fail score of 16 and a maximum weighted score of 80.

5. The weighted score can be broken down into several error categories. The categories, their symbols, and the number of their instances in the test are: color adjectives (C, 54 instances), shape nouns (S, 53), size adjectives (I, 12), verbs (V, 16), spatial prepositions (P, 7) and other prepositions, conjunctions and adverbs (A, 21). C, S, and I together constitute the class of "references." Each of the categories is tallied separately for research purposes.

6. Some instructions (marked with a † or a ‡) contain references which are repeated from an earlier part of the same (†) or the previous (‡) instruction. These should be read "neutrally," that is with no stress to indicate the relationship—each phrase is read as if it is new or first. For research purposes any of the instructions which contain or prepare for repetitions and were performed incorrectly can be repeated with the correct intonation at the end of the test (in addition to the immediate repetition described in Section 2).

B. *Weighted Scoring*

1. Credit is not obtainable from "passive" items such as one of the two optional phrases in Instruction 28, the antecedent phrase of the conditional in Instruction 31, and the negated phrase in Instructions 37 and 38.

2. In Parts A-E of the test, the initial verb is "show me" or "take." These should not be scored and should be demonstrated if erroneously performed. In Part F of the test, "putting on" and "picking up" are acceptable responses for "touch" but not conversely.

3. Perseverations, that is, manipulation of clearly additional items to those specified in the instructions when the instruction itself has been performed correctly, are scored as errors in the "pass-fail" system but do not affect weighted scores.

*Instruction 25.* "Next to" is accepted for "behind."

*Instruction 26.* The red square has to be the agent for scoring "with" as correct. "Put on" is accepted for "touch with".

*Instruction 27.* "With" is not accepted for "and.."

*Instruction 28.* Exclusive but no inclusive interpretation of the conjunction "or" is correct. If two chips are manipulated, then "or" is scored as an error and only the phrase yielding higher credit is scored, even if the verb is misinterpreted as one requiring two references (e.g., "put ... on ..."). In the latter case, the verb is scored as an error.

*Instruction 30.* "On top of" and "next to" are accepted for "in front of" but "under" is not.

*Instruction 31.* "Black circle" is not scored. If a chip is manipulated, an error is recorded on "if" and the last verb and reference are scored. Correct abstaining from manipulation receives a weighted score of 4 for consistency.

*Instruction 32.* "Squares" receives credit if at least two are manipulated (cf. Instructions 34 and 36). "All" receives credit if and only if all chips of a single category are manipulated. "One" receives credit if precisely one chip is excluded from the manipulated class. "The" receives credit if precisely one whole class is manipulated (cf. Instruction 36).

*Instruction 33.* "Next to," "on top of," and "under" are accepted for "beside."

*Instruction 35.* "Between" is accepted as correct along any of the three dimensions in Euclidean Space.

*Instruction 37.* If the red circle is manipulated, then "no" should be scored as an error for a weighted score of 3. Otherwise, score "no" as correct and assume the subject intended the final reference and score it even if he manipulated a red chip or a circle.

*Instruction 38.* Same as Instruction 37 with "instead of" substituted for "no" and "white square" substituted for "red circle."

C. *Summary of Weighted Scores*

| Item | Code | Number of occurrences |
| --- | --- | --- |
| Parts A–E | | |
| Shape nouns | S | 26 |
| Color adjectives | C | 29 |
| Size adjectives | I | 12 |
| Total references | | 67 |
| Part F | | |
| Shape nouns | S | 27 |
| Color adjectives | C | 25 |
| Verbs | V | 16 |
| Spatial prepositions | P | 7 |
| Particles | A | 21 |
| Total references | | 52 |
| Total weighted score | | 96 |
| Whole test (Parts A–F) | | |
| Shape nouns | S | 53 |
| Color adjectives | C | 54 |
| Size adjectives | I | 12 |
| Verbs | V | 16 |
| Spatial prepositions | P | 7 |
| Particles | A | 21 |
| Total references | | 125 |
| Total weighted score | | 163 |

D. *Summary of Pass-Fail Scores*
   Parts A-E            23
   Part F               16
   Whole test (Parts A-F)   39

## *Token Test.*

A. Present tokens in a random order. Instructions may be repeated       Maximum Points
   once
       1. *Show me a* **circle**                                    1
           S
       2. *Show me a* **square**                                    1
           S
       3. *Show me a* **yellow** *one*                              1
           C
       4. *Show me a* **red** *one*                                 1
           C
       5. *Show me a* **blue** *one*                                1
           C
   * 6. *Show me a* **green** *one*                                                    1
           C
       7. *Show me a* **white** *one*                               1
           C
                                         TOTAL   A(7)

B. Present only large tokens. Instructions may be repeated once
       8. *Show me the* **yellow square**                           2
       9. *Show me the* **blue circle**                             2
   * 10. *Show me the* **green circle**                                                2
       11. *Show me the* **white square**                           2
           C     S
                                  TOTAL   B(8)

C. Present all tokens. Do not repeat instructions
   * 12. *Show me the* **small white circle**                                          3
       13. *Show me the* **large yellow square**                    3
       14. *Show me the* **large green square**                     3
       15. *Show me the* **small blue square**                      3
           I    C    S
                                  TOTAL   C(12)

D. Present large tokens only. Do not repeat instructions
   * 16. *Take the* **red circle** *and the* **green square**                          4
   †* 17. *Take the* **yellow square** *and the* **blue square**                       4
       18. *Take the* **white square** *and the* **green circle**   4
   †* 19. *Take the* **white circle** *and the* **red circle**                         4
           C    S          C    S
                                  TOTAL   D(16)

E. Present all tokens. Do not repeat instructions
   * 20. *Take the* **large white circle** *and the* **small green square**            6
   * 21. *Take the* **small blue circle** *and the* **large yellow square**            6

† * 22. *Take the* **large green square** *and the* **large red square**     6
† * 23. *Take the* **large white square** *and the* **small green circle**     6
            I    C    S         I    C    S

                                 TOTAL E(24)

F. Present large tokens only. Do not repeat instructions
    * 24. **Put** *the* **red circle on** *the* **green square**     6
         V    C    S    P      C    S
     25. **Put** *the* **white square behind** *the* **yellow circle**     6
         V    C    S    P      C    S
    * 26. **Touch** *the* **blue circle with** *the* **red square**     6
         V     C    S    P    C    S
   ‡ * 27. **Touch** *the* **blue circle and** *the* **red square**     6
         V     C    S    A    C    S

   ‡ 28. **Pick up** *the* $\begin{pmatrix} \text{blue circle} \\ \text{C} \quad \text{S} \end{pmatrix}$ or *the* $\begin{pmatrix} \text{red square} \\ \text{C} \quad \text{S} \end{pmatrix}$     4
         V                  A

† * 29. **Move** *the* **green square away from** *the* **yellow square**     6
         V    C    S      P      C    S
     30. **Put** *the* **white circle in front of** *the* **blue square**     6
         V    C    S      P      C    S
     31. **If** *there is a black circle,* **pick up** *the* **red square**     4
         A               V    C    S
     32. **Pick up all the squares except** *the* **yellow one**     7
            V   A   A    S      A      C    A
    * 33. **Put** *the* **green square beside** *the* **red circle**     6
         V    C    S    P      C    S
     34. **Touch all the squares slowly and all the circles quickly**     10
         V   A   A    S      A    A   A    S      A
† * 35. **Put** *the* **red circle between** *the* **yellow square** *and the*     8
         V    C    S    P      C
         **green square**

     36. **Touch all the circles, except** *the* **green one**     7
         V   A   A    S      A      C    A
     37. **Pick up** *the* *red circle* -**no**— the **white square**     4
         V           A      C    S
   ‡ 38. **Instead of** *the white square,* **pick up** *the* **yellow circle**     4
         A               V      C    S
   ‡ 39. **Together with** *the* **yellow circle, pick up** *the* **blue circle**     6
         A       C    S     V      C    S

                                 TOTAL F(96)

# 11

## Lesions Underlying Defective Performances on the Token Test: A CT Scan Study

LUIGI A. VIGNOLO

There is a consensus that lateralized and focal lesions can be associated with impairments of auditory comprehension. What is less clear is the precise extent and location of these lesions. Most authors agree that such lesions tend to be located in, or in the vicinity of, the left superior temporal gyrus, but the crucial area for comprehension is still a matter of dispute (Bogen & Bogen, 1976).

In 1874, Wernicke identified the area associated with auditory comprehension without qualification as the first temporal convolution. Other authors extended it to the entire posterior language zone, that is, to a large temporo-parietal region, or else to the posterior half of the first (and second) temporal convolutions. Perhaps the majority of recent researchers restrict the area to the posterior third of the first temporal gyrus. Such disagreement represents a good reason for looking further into this question.

## MATERIALS AND METHODS

We have had the opportunity to investigate this problem in 90 patients with cerebrovascular accidents (CVA), who were referred to our

Aphasia Unit for evaluation, because they were thought to suffer from a left (dominant) hemisphere lesion.

*Auditory verbal comprehension* was assessed by means of the 36-item version of the Token Test. Scores were corrected for educational level according to the criteria established by De Renzi (Chapter 3 of this volume). Patients who scored 10 or less (out of 36) were arbitrarily judged to have a severe comprehension deficit, those scoring 20 to 29 were judged to have a mild deficit and above 29, no deficit. Two patients with marked color agnosia were excluded.

*The site and extent of the lesion* were evaluated by means of an EMI-scanner CT 1000 with water bag. Basic information about the CT scan is available in the original papers by Hounsfield (1973) and Ambrose (1973). In essence, a CT machine yields a series of x-ray pictures of the brain, corresponding to different horizontal sections. As more than 300,000 x-ray beams, 2–4 mm, are aimed through the head, they provide information about the density of the structures they have encountered. Therefore each section shows some of the main structures of the brain, differentiated according to density. Cerebrovascular lesions can be visualized as areas of either hypodensity (infarcts and old hemorrhages) or hyperdensity (recent hemorrhages). A standard procedure yields eight 13 mm horizontal sections of the brain; an enhanced procedure involves injection of contrast material before the scan. Only lesions without enhancement were studied. The contour of the lesion was traced on each section and then mapped on a lateral diagram of the hemisphere, according to the procedure described by Mazzocchi and Vignolo (1978). In essence, the procedure has two steps: The first establishes the angle of the CT section, and the second transfers the picture of the lesion on to the standard lateral diagram. Composite contour maps were then drawn following the procedure described by Howes and Boller (1975).

The *time-since-lesion* is an important parameter in establishing the correlation between the Token Test scores and the lesion. Patients were divided into 3 groups, according to the interval between stroke, on the one hand, and Token Test and CT scan, on the other:

1. *Acute* group: both Token Test and CT scan from 2 days to 3 weeks post-onset.
2. *Recent* group: Token Test between 3 weeks and 2 months, CT scan after more than 3 weeks.
3. *Late* group: Token Test and CT after more than 2 months post-onset.

The best group for correlation is the *recent* group because, between 3 weeks and 2 months, edema and transient blood-flow changes surrounding the lesion have disappeared, diaschisis presumably has vanished, and functional compensation from contralateral or adjacent areas has not yet set in. As a consequence, auditory-verbal comprehension deficits reflect the extent of the underlying lesion more faithfully at this stage than at earlier or later stages post-onset.

In this report, attention will be focused exclusively on patients examined between 21 and 60 days post-onset, that is, during the optimal period for correlation. This group was composed of 44 patients with lesions in the left (dominant) hemisphere.

## RESULTS AND DISCUSSION

In order to find the locus of lesion specifically associated with poor comprehension, we singled out patients with Token Test scores $\leq 10$ and patients with Token Test scores $\geq 20$, and then compared the lesions in the 2 groups.

The first group (with low Token Test scores) included 17 patients. Scores ranged from 0 to 8, and the mean was 3.6 points. Five had very large lesions involving both the anterior (prerolandic) and the posterior (postrolandic) areas of the convexity of the left hemisphere, as well as some deeper structures. Figure 11.1 shows a composite lateral map of the lesions in these 5 cases. Contours do not indicate the individual lesions, but the degree of overlapping of lesions. Thus the outer region includes all the areas that are damaged by 1 lesion only, while the inner region indicates the area damaged by all 5 lesions. The frequency of involvement of some deep structures which cannot be visualized on a diagram of the convexity, such as the insula (I), the lenticular nucleus (L) and the internal capsule (IC) is shown in the upper right hand corner of the figure. The insula is the most frequently damaged structure, being involved in 4 cases. The next most frequently damaged is the lenticular nucleus (involved in 3 cases), while only 2 lesions go as deep as the internal capsule. These lesions are too large to be definitive; they suggest merely that the critical area for comprehension is to be found somewhere in the perisylvian region.

Somewhat more precise information can be obtained by investigating less extensive lesions. Consideration will next be given to cases with medium-sized lesions, that is, lesions involving a surface area between 2 and 40 cm$^2$ including damage to some underlying deep structures.

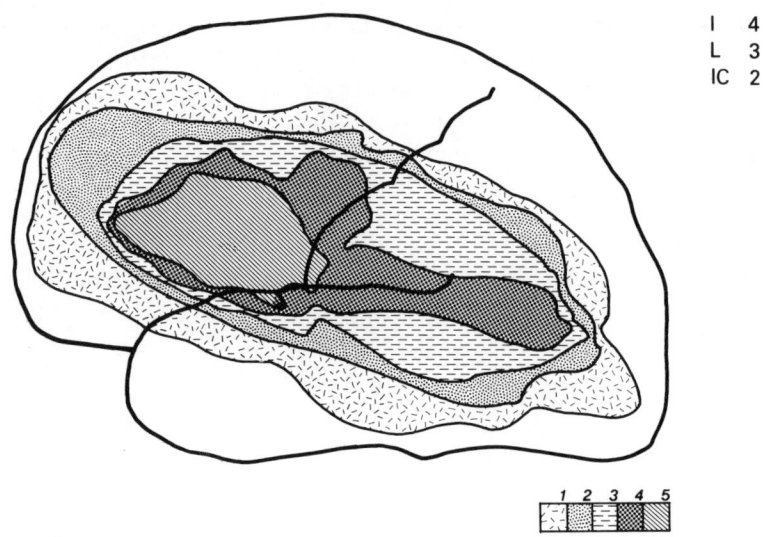

**FIGURE 11.1.** *Composite lateral contour map of large lesions in 5 patients with low Token Test scores. I = insula, L = lenticular nucleus, IC = internal capsule.*

There were 10 such cases in our series. The lesions were predominantly postrolandic in 5 patients, predominantly prerolandic in 3, and perirolandic in 2. However, as shown in Figure 11.2, the area of greatest overlap (9 lesions out of 10) was located approximately between the middle and the posterior thirds of the first temporal convolution. In depth, the anterior insula was damaged in 5 cases—which also involved the lenticular nucleus and, in one instance, the internal capsule—while in the other 5 cases the lesions merely impinged on the posterior insula. In 2 other cases with medium-sized lesions, the damage was confined to the deep structures, that is, the insula, the lenticular nucleus and, in one case, the internal capsule as well, as shown in Figure 11.3.

In summary, the lesions associated with low Token Test scores were either extensive, rather uninformative lesions (5 cases out of 17); or medium-sized lesions (10 superficial *and* deep, and 2 deep *only*). This suggests that the critical areas in which damage is associated with poor comprehension comprise a small region between the middle and the posterior thirds of the first temporal convolution, and the underlying insular and subcortical structures.

If this indication is correct, that is, if the areas of greatest overlap shown in Figures 11.2 and 11.3 indeed correspond to crucial loci for auditory-verbal comprehension, then lesions associated with *good* auditory comprehension should either spare them or damage them only

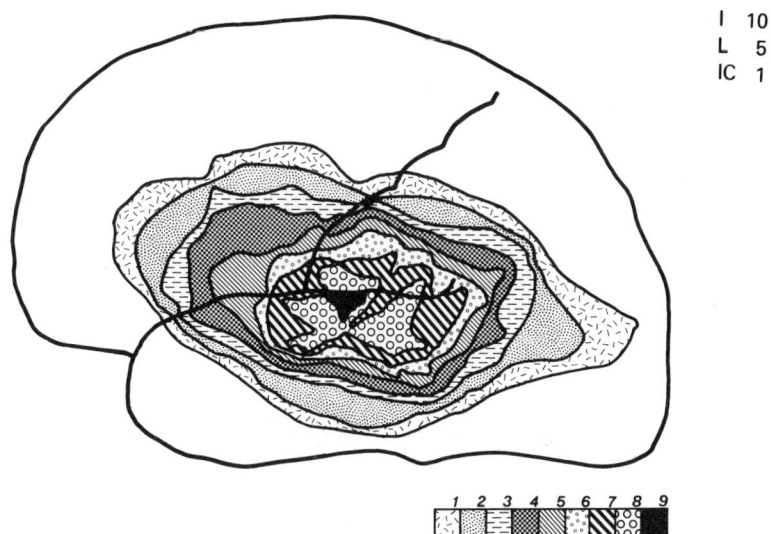

**FIGURE 11.2.** *Composite lateral contour map of medium-sized lesions in 10 patients with low Token Test scores.*

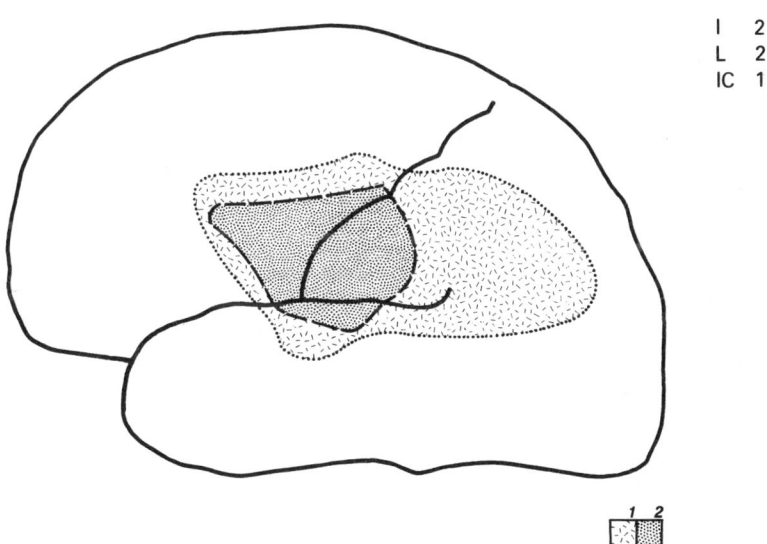

**FIGURE 11.3.** *Composite lateral contour map of medium-sized lesions confined to the deep structures in 2 patients with low Token Test scores.*

lightly. In order to verify this, the lesions in patients with Token Test scores ≥ 20 were examined. Fourteen such patients were found. Mean Token Test score was 25.2 with a range from 20 to 35. Since the normal cut-off score of the Token Test is 29 it would suggest that though auditory-verbal comprehension in some of these patients was not entirely unimpaired, it was only a mild impairment. The damage was superficial in 7 cases and deep in 5, while in 2 cases no lesions could be detected on the CT sections.

The contour map of the 7 superficial lesions is shown in Figure 11.4. Compared with those associated with low Token Test scores, these lesions were smaller and more scattered (maximum overlap is 3 lesions out of 7, versus 9 out of 10 in the poor comprehension group), and they involved the deeper structures less often. Most of them were clearly marginal with respect to those associated with poor comprehension. The "critical" area in the posterior first temporal convolution was not entirely spared, but was damaged partially and much less frequently.

As to the lesions confined to the deep structures, in the 5 patients with good comprehension they were limited to the internal capsule or to the anterior insula, that is, they were placed either more deeply or more anteriorly than those of patients with poor comprehension.

In conclusion, these comparisons constitute an initial report which supports the notion that the crucial area for auditory-verbal comprehen-

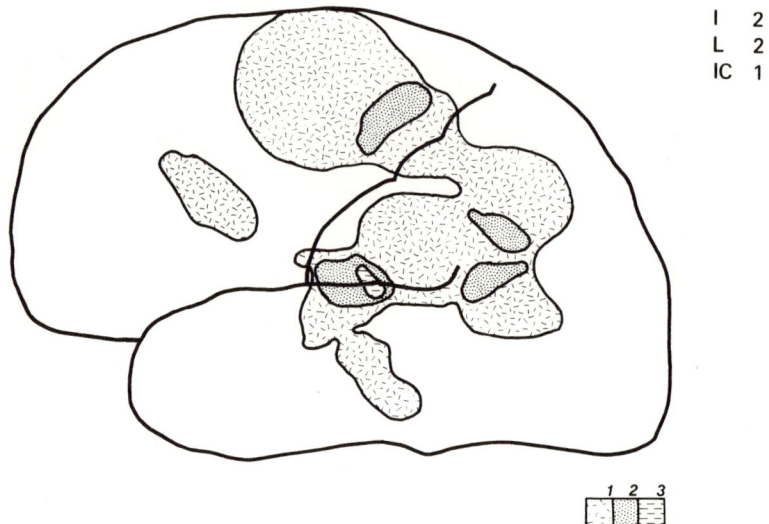

**FIGURE 11.4.** *Composite lateral contour map of seven superficial lesions in patients with high Token Test scores.*

sion (as measured by the Token Test scores) is located between the middle and the posterior thirds of the first temporal gyrus, encroaching upon the posterior insula region. It is also suggested that damage confined to the left posterior insula and to the surrounding deep structures may impair comprehension. What must next be established, then, is the level of Token Test performance in a large group of patients with small, circumscribed, focal lesions.

## ACKNOWLEDGMENT

I wish to thank Dr. Alessandra Macchi for her help in the preparation of this chapter.

# VI
## RESEARCH DIRECTIONS

# 12

## Epilogue: Research Applications and Directions

MAUREEN DENNIS

The vitality of the Token Test after 16 years can be seen in the breadth of its applications: an assessment procedure with adult aphasics; a means of assessing language change after therapy; a yardstick for language development in childhood aphasics; and a means of testing the language competence of selected parts of the brain. The diversity of a test's uses is not, however, a measure of its power as a test. How well does the Token Test measure the language functions it was designed to assess, and how reliably does it discriminate groups with different types of language pathology and/or brain damage?

To answer such questions, it is necessary to evaluate both what has been learned about the Token Test and what is yet to be established. We will review the properties of the Token Test (the linguistic functions in its items, the cognitive skills to which test performance is related); the range of its applications (the manner of its uses, its scoring systems); its discriminative power (its capacity to separate groups differing on other language measures and its value in capturing commonality between different language pathologies); and its status as the behavioral anchor of a clinico-pathological correlation (can it discriminate different lesion loci?).

## THE PROPERTIES OF THE TOKEN TEST

The Token Test consists of a series of nonredundant oral commands cast in a variety of linguistic modes. The diversity of the test items simplifies interpretation of proficient performance but makes ambiguous the meaning of a test impairment. While a high score is a sign that many different sentence structures have been understood, a low score does not indicate which of the several test attributes was not processed; information, syntactic variation, or particular syntactic forms. For this reason, it is important to consider how performance varies with the requirements of the test.

One technique is to analyze the set of linguistic structures contained in the test items, so that the microstructure of the individual items can be described. The linguistic features studied in this manner are word frequency, Length–Complexity Index, and semantic case relationships (Whitaker & Noll, 1972; Whitaker & Selnes, 1978; Whitaker & Whitaker, this volume). These analyses have provided formal descriptions of the intra- and interitem diversity in the Token Test; and, more important, have refined the concepts of test ambiguity and test complexity. Ambiguity arises because some command forms permit two readings, and, hence, two equally correct responses. Complexity in the test is a result of either increased noun phrase loading (Parts III and IV relative to Parts I and II) or greater structural complexity (Part V).

To provide a formalism for the linguistic structures in the test is not, of itself, to predict how such structures will affect comprehension performance; and, in fact, there has been little attempt to manipulate the role of the test properties in actual performance. Studies which reduce the item variance by omitting some command forms and/or token properties (e.g., Mack & Boller, this volume) serve the useful function of making the test more homogeneous (and hence, in some instances, more interpretable), but do not address the issue of how each type of coordinate or syntactic complexity in the test contributes to the ability to execute the commands.

What has not been evaluated is the effect on performance of one aspect of complexity (e.g., a particular syntactic form) while holding constant the other component of difficulty (e.g., the information level of the coordinate structures of the item noun phrases). Nor has the role of structural ambiguity on performance been assessed. Many locative prepositions in the Token Test permit several different spatial realizations, depending on the topographic reference point the subject takes; the preposition "with" can mark an instrumental case or a deleted coordinate structure. In general, the coordinate structures of Parts I–IV represent a more homogeneous form of difficulty than the syntactically complex structures of Part V, which make demands on diverse syntactic processing. How each type of syntactic complexity affects performance is not clear.

Unresolved issues of the nature and distribution of difficulty in the Token Test have obscured an evaluation of the role of other cognitive skills in test performance. This is seen in the issue of short-term memory. Although the Token Test presupposes a degree of intactness of short-term memory processes, it is not clear how memory interacts with stimulus and response demands of the test to determine the level of performance.

Applied in its most simple form, a short-term memory interpretation of Token Test performance would imply a view of language as a finite-state Markov process, with difficulty being a simple function of the length of the commands. The reasons for questioning this view are both logical and empirical. While conceivably true for the coordinate structures, this cannot hold in those instances where complexity is effected by syntactic features such as embeddings, so that a relatively short command may be more difficult to process than a longer but structurally more simple item. The data suggest that test difficulty is not uniformly a result of either the length of the command or of syntactic difficulty, but, instead, varies with the kind of deficit under consideration. Developmental dysphasics have great difficulty with the coordinate structures in the test (Part IV), although their performance actually improves when the difficulty in Part V becomes structural or grammatical (Tallal, 1975). Infantile hemiplegic children missing the left hemisphere, by contrast, fail on the syntactically complex section of the test (Part V), but are quite proficient at the most difficult Part IV coordinate structures (Dennis & Whitaker, 1976).

Some subjects fail because of both syntactic and information demands of the Test (e.g., Noll & Randolph, 1978). It is those instances in which the two types of complexity are dissociated that most obviously resist a unitary memory explanation.

Even when it is evident that coordinate complexity is the main cause of failure on the test, it is not clear whether a perceptual problem—concerning the rate of processing acoustic material—or a mnemonic deficit is involved. The plausibility of a particular interpretation is generally enhanced when some independent evidence exists in the same subjects for related deficits. For example, the observation that childhood dysphasics execute only the last part of Token Test commands (Tallal, 1975) is consistent with other evidence that they are impaired in analyzing rapid streams of acoustic information.

The relationship between Token Test performance and independent measures of memory is uncertain. Some studies report such findings; others do not. Aside from the conflicting results, the reasoning behind some of the comparisons made to test the memory hypothesis can be questioned. Lesser (1976) correlated sequence memory tests (for auditory–verbal, visual–verbal, and gestural material) with the number of information units (for content words and attributes) in the Token Test. Order is irrelevant to all the coordinate structures in the Test; nor does linear order seem to be involved in many of the Part V syntactic structures. It is not clear, therefore, why sequence memory would be a predictor of the number of units of information correctly executed, and it is not surprising that the asymmetrical distribution of errors in the Token Test, Part V, does not correlate with such units of information (Whitaker & Selnes, 1978).

A more basic problem concerns the interpretation of test intercorrelations. Cognitive tests, especially those involving the same stimulus modality, often correlate with each other. The meaning of this is not obvious. Of themselves, correlations do not signal how two items are processed, and hence, whether they are causally related. The demonstration of a correlation between two tests means, in effect, that the same individuals pass or fail the upper and lower bounds. This may be either because the tests tap a common process or else because a more severe form of a given disorder impairs a whole range of performances, including the two measured. When Token Test scores are found to correlate with a whole series of tests, the latter interpretation is the more probable. If a pattern of intertest correlation and dissociation can be shown, however, it becomes more likely that the observed correlation represents common processing rather than global deficit.

It is difficult to make a clear statement of the role of memory in Token Test performance because many of the appropriate studies have not been done. Studying the relationship between memory for different components of an utterance (content, linear order, syntactic structure) and the appropriate parts of the Token Test would establish the specificity of the memory processes operating in performance. Asking the subjects to repeat or otherwise identify the commands before executing them would clarify the respective roles of perceptual processing and short-term memory in Token Test performance. Evaluation of any discrepancy between production and discrimination of complex commands would serve to decide between memory registration and retrieval explanations.

The role of the stimulus modality and the processing pattern has been addressed in part. Poeck and Hartje (this volume) found that aphasics are similarly impaired on written and oral versions of the Token Test. These data make less plausible a simple memory interpretation, in the sense that the written version makes fewer memory demands than the oral form. What is unclear is how each of the modality and the processing patterns produce performance in isolation. Oral information is auditory and patterned in time. Written information is visual and patterned in space. In changing both together, it becomes difficult to assess the role of each in isolation. A comparison of written Token Test performance given in the normal manner with a written version in which words are paced as they are in speech would provide useful information about how the processing pattern normally used with auditory information contributes to memory for and execution of the commands.

There is no doubt that the Token Test draws on other cognitive skills, among them short-term memory. In this sense, a severe mental impairment, in memory or in some other function, will cause test failure. Nevertheless, it is not the case that memory deficits are a universal explanation for test disruptions.

In short, the Token Test is complex. The lack of redundancy in the message and the absence of contextual cues to meaning do not, of themselves, entail that language processing be simple. An analysis of the intra- and interitem properties of the Test reveals that it contains two independent components of difficulty. What remains to be established is how each facet of test complexity draws on cognitive skills such as short-term memory to produce the observed levels of test performance.

## RANGE OF TOKEN TEST APPLICATIONS

The Token Test may be considered as a variable in an experiment. In one set of studies, it is the measure by which the effects of other factors are judged (i.e., the dependent variable); in another, it is the dimension whose operation is indexed by other measures or subject groupings (i.e., the independent variable).

The first application is more common. By taking language status and/or side of brain damage as the independent variables, one can create subject groupings (e.g., aphasic–nonaphasic, fluent–nonfluent, left-damaged–right-damaged) and ask whether these groupings are reflected in Token Test scores. Although this has proved a productive use of the test, some important issues have been rarely addressed, and the scoring methods have sometimes limited the possible range of interpretations of the results.

The independent variables chosen in studies of the first type have generally represented prevailing interest areas (e.g., the fluency–nonfluency dimension of aphasia). Other aspects of brain damage have been largely ignored, despite the fact that they are of central importance to the clinical picture in aphasia. Thus, for example, there is no information about the role of lesion etiology and lesion duration in Token Test performance. Both aspects of brain damage are indirectly represented in the literature (e.g., in studies of recovery), but their particular contribution to the level of performance is unclear. It would be desirable to have an independent assessment of the specific role of lesion age comparable to, for example, Fitzhugh, Fitzhugh, and Reitan's (1962) studies of the effect of the same factor on verbal intelligence. By collapsing across the dimensions of lesion etiology and lesion duration, significant information may have been obscured.

The manner in which the Token Test scores are analyzed has, in some instances, failed to maximize the discriminative power of the test. Individuals may fail a complex test for different reasons, so that a total score will not necessarily capture the diversity of the processing failures. As a result, the inferences which can be drawn when the test scores are the dependent variable depend upon how much is extracted from the scores. This is sometimes the least detailed aspect of a study. Most studies employ the dimensions of brain damage in a dichotomous manner (e.g., the fluent–nonfluent distinction); indeed, some dimensions are difficult to consider in other than a categorical way (e.g., right-damaged–left-damaged). The independent variable, in short, is often a dichotomous one. When the measure is also dichotomous (as, for example, in the case of cut-off scores), then the only information which can be captured is that at the intersection of the two categories.

Techniques for gaining more information about test performance include a list of critical items and an error analysis. Listing the items which language-disordered subjects fail is one means of deriving hypotheses about the reasons for failure, although it does not test those hypotheses: The critical item list indicates which commands are most difficult, but it does not signal the kind of processing that the subjects have failed to perform. An error analysis can be a valuable supplement to whole-score test analyses. However, in some instances it is not possible to pinpoint the type of error in an unambiguous way. In addition, some parts of the test demand increased attention to one type of processing and may thus cause a deterioration in another operation which, without the overload, could normally be performed. Furthermore, in performing an error analysis on the items in Part V, chance performance is maximized. To use the error analysis directly as an index of specific types of processing is to suppose nonrandom performance on each erroneous item, a shaky assumption when there is only one item of each type and a finite probability of the correct token being selected. Failure on any single test item such as "Touch the blue circle with the red square" may represent a processing failure for commands with an Object-Instrument order of constituents, but it may, equally, represent a failure in any one of a variety of unrelated processes. Because this is the only instance in the test of that particular construction, it is important that it not be overinterpreted. In any event, a selective syntactic deficit would not be reflected in a total error score. An error analysis should be a beginning, a source of clues for creating experimental tests to pinpoint the processing deficits.

The use of Token Test scores as a dichotomous independent variable, although a less common application, has so far proved fruitful. Vignolo (this volume) subdivides aphasics on the basis of Token Test scores, and uses as the dependent variable the extent and locus of lesion. In this manner, a dichotomous variable—Token Test scores—is matched against a finely grained analysis of lesion properties.

Perhaps it is the case that either the dependent variable, the independent variable, or both, should be amenable to some form of detailed analysis. Significant information may be lost if both the factors to be assessed and the measures themselves are dichotomous.

## DISCRIMINATIVE POWER

Broadly, the Token Test has been used to group subjects in two different ways; first, as a means of separating individuals shown to be at different points on a behavioral continuum; second, as a technique for establishing commonalities of performance between otherwise diverse subject populations.

The burden of the first approach has concerned whether the Token Test can discriminate between groups labeled "fluent" and "nonfluent" on the basis of other aspects of language performance. The results have generally proved to be contradictory. The reasons for this concern both the subject selection and the test scoring systems.

The categorization fluent-nonfluent refers to relative standing with respect to language production. The comprehension performance of the two groups is not so readily separable. At least some aspects of comprehension are impaired in nonfluent aphasics. Zurif, Caramazza, and Myerson (1972), for example, demonstrated a deficit in the tacit comprehension of grammatical structures in these subjects. In light of such findings, it is not surprising that other measures of comprehension such as the Token Test often fail to reveal a clear separation between the two groups. Token Test deficits are correlated with the severity of receptive, but not expressive, impairments (Kreindler, Gheorghita, & Voinescu, 1971), suggesting that whether or not Token Test scores differentiate fluent from nonfluent aphasics may depend largely on the comprehension status of the nonfluent group.

When a difference is found, its nature depends on how the test is scored. If global or whole-test score is used, any difference will be a quantitative one. With a more fine-grained analysis, both qualitative and quantitative differences may be apparent. Mack and Boller (this volume) report that fluent and nonfluent aphasics can be differentiated by both the number of lexical errors (a difference of degree) and the relative proportion of syntactic errors (a difference of kind). These data suggest that there are some processing differences in Token Test performance discriminating fluent and nonfluent aphasics not wholly attributable to extralinguistic factors like memory (Zaidel, this volume). Whether these differences are demonstrable, however, depends on the level of analysis.

If the problem of interpreting correlations is pertinent to any consideration of the relationship between the Token Test and other measures of cognition, it becomes critical in the second application of the Token Test, inferring functional similarities between diverse groups. This issue has been studied in the context of the regression hypothesis, which is the proposal that the language dissolution of adult aphasics can best be described as a relapse to an earlier stage of language development. The Token Test has been used to study the parallel between the patterns of early language acquisition and those of adult aphasic breakdown, in the hope that such analogues will show whether similar rules operate in the acquisition and breakdown of language.

There is reasonably good correlation between the rank errors of children and adult aphasics (Whitaker & Selnes, 1978), but little concordance for error distribution. The Token Test items which reveal most age variance account for only one-third of aphasic errors (Poeck, Orgass, Kerschensteiner, & Hartje, 1974).

Even the parallels which correlations demonstrate mean only that dimensions like linguistic complexity operate for most language users. One could readily construct a Token Test in such a manner as to produce a perfect correlation between child and aphasic performances. The first items of such a test would involve discrimination of circles and squares in response to the spoken commands, "circle" and "square"; the final items would drastically overload both the coordinate and syntactic processing capacity of both groups (e.g., "Touch the small blue square, using both the large white circle and the small red square next to the small yellow circle, after I touch the large green circle"). A high correlation between child and aphasic scores, in this instance, would mean only that dimensions of difficulty operate for both groups of language users. More than a correlation is needed in order to conclude that a similarity of processing operations is involved.

## CLINICO-PATHOLOGICAL CORRELATIONS

The issue of whether fluent and nonfluent aphasics can be discriminated has typically been addressed by considering the relationship between two behavioural measures. In one sense, then, any correlation between Token Test scores and typologies like fluent-nonfluent aphasia is circular. Because they are both ways of classifying language—specifically, auditory comprehension—it would be surprising if they were not related. Of themselves, these studies do not address directly the relation between language status and defined brain damage.

The concept of nonfluent or Broca's aphasia, for example, is a hybrid, being a cross between an anatomical and a functional description. Nonfluent aphasics generally have anteriorly located lesions, but the diagnosis is primarily a functional one. Thus, "Broca's aphasia" refers more to a type of language than to a lesion in the third frontal convolution in the left hemisphere. As a result, the type and extent of brain damage underlying a particular aphasia is often unclear, and the lesions themselves may differ so that, for example, nonfluent aphasias encompass a wider area of damage than fluent aphasias (De Renzi, this volume).

It is of importance, then, to consider the relationship between Token Test performance and known brain damage, and, hence, whether the Token Test can be used in any equation relating language function to specific brain pathologies. This has been addressed in two ways. In the first, a dimension of known brain damage is selected and the question asked whether Token Test scores differ according to the dimension. In the second, Test scores are the basis of categorizing subjects and the issue is whether brain damage varies systematically with this categorization.

Reports of the first kind have confirmed that a hemispheric asymmetry exists for auditory comprehension as measured by the Token Test. Those studies which place Token Test scores in the context of other language measures have generally been able to go beyond a simple demonstration of left hemisphere-right hemisphere differences to a beginning account of the processing characteristics of each cerebral hemisphere (e.g., Zaidel, this volume). The second type of analysis has been directed towards describing the characteristics of Token Test impairment within the left hemisphere (e.g., Vignolo, this volume). In general, the use of the Token Test in clinico-pathological correlations has revealed that it is not sensitive to cerebral damage in general, but instead, is affected by the side of brain damage and, to some extent, by the within-hemisphere damage in the left hemisphere. It is the latter question—how the Token Test scores vary with damage to the language areas of the left hemisphere—which remains to be fully answered.

## CONCLUSIONS

The Token Test is robust, and it has demonstrated its applicability in diverse settings. Our knowledge of the test, however, is wide rather than deep: While we know much about the range of its use, we can formalize rather little about the nature of the language processing it signals. Perhaps it is now time to stop extending its range in favor of beginning to use the new technical information—analyses of the linguistic properties of the test items and the nonlinguistic determinants of performance—to discover how the test measures language in groups to which it has already been administered.

## ACKNOWLEDGMENT

Preparation of this chapter was supported by Ontario Mental Health Foundation Individual Award Grant No. 704 and a Research Scholarship to the author.

# References

Aaronson, D. Stimulus factors and listening strategies in auditory memory: A theoretical analysis. *Cognitive Psychology,* 1974, *6,* 108-132.

Adler, S. Social class bases of language: A reexamination of socioeconomic, sociopsychological, and sociolinguistic factors. *Journal of the American Speech and Hearing Association,* 1973, *15,* 3-9.

Albert, M. L. Short-term memory and aphasia. *Brain and Language,* 1976, *3,* 28-33.

Ambrose, J. Computerized transverse axial scanning (tomography). Part 2. Clinical application. *British Journal of Radiology,* 1973, *46,* 1023-1047.

Ballet, G., & Laignel, L. Aphasie. In Bronardel & Gilbert (Eds.) *Nouveau traité de médecine* (Vol. 31, *Sémiologie Nerveuse*). Paris: 1911.

Benton, A. L. The measurement of aphasic disorders. In *Aspectos patologicos del lenguaje.* Actas de las Primeras Jornadas Internacionales del Lenguaje. Lima, Peru, 1973. Pp. 61-78.

Bernstein, B. *Class, Codes and Control* (2nd ed.). New York: Schocken Books, 1974.

Berry, W. R. A psychometric reconsideration of the Token Test. Paper presented at the Third Annual Conference in Clinical Aphasiology, Albuquerque, N. M., 1975.

Boder, E. Developmental dyslexia: Prevailing diagnostic concepts and a new diagnostic approach. *Progress in Learning Disabilities,* 1971, *2,* 293-321.

Bogen, J. E., & Bogen, G. M. Wernicke's region: Where is it? *Annals of the New York Academy of Sciences,* 1976, *280,* 834-843.

Bogen, J. E., Kumar, S., Johnson, T., Ozgur, M., Smith, A., Thale, M., Witton, R., & Zaidel, E. Ventricular shunting for hydrocephalus after hemispherectomy. Submitted for publication, 1978. (Abstract)

Bogen, J. E., & Vogel, P. J. Neurologic status in the long term following complete cerebral commissurotomy. In F. Michel & B. Schott (Eds.), *Les syndromes de disconnexion calleuse chez l'homme.* Lyon: Hôpital Neurologique, 1975.

Boller, F. Latent aphasia: Right and left "non-aphasic" brain-damaged patients compared. *Cortex*, 1968, *4*, 245-256.

Boller, F. Comprehension disorders in aphasia: A historical review. *Brain and Language*, 1978, *5*, 149-165.

Boller F., Kim, Y., & Mack, J. L. Auditory comprehension in aphasia. In H. Whitaker & H. Whitaker (Eds.), *Studies in Neurolinguistics* (Vol. 3). New York: Academic Press, 1977.

Boller, F., & Vignolo, L. A. Latent sensory aphasia in hemisphere-damaged patients: An experimental study with the Token Test. *Brain*, 1966, *89*, 815-830.

Bortolini, U., Tagliavini, C., & Zampolli, A. *Lessico di Frequenza della Lingua Italiana.* Garzanti, Milano, 1972.

Clark, H. H., & Clark, E. V. *Psychology and Language.* New York: Harcourt Brace Jovanovich, 1977.

Cohen, R., Kelter, S., Engel, D., List, G., & Strohner, H. Zur Validität des Token Tests. *Der Nervenarzt*, 1976, *47*, 357-361.

Cohen, R., Kelter, S., & Schäfer, B. Zum Einfluss des Sprachverständnisse auf die Leistungen im Token Test. *Zeitschrift für Klinische Psychologie*, 1977, *6*, 1-14.

Curtiss, S. *Genie. A Psycholinguistic Study of Modern-Day "Wild Child."* New York: Academic Press, 1977.

Dennis, M., & Whitaker, H. A. Language acquisition following hemidecortication: Linguistic superiority of the left over the right hemisphere. *Brain and Language*, 1976, *3*, 404-433.

De Renzi, E. Un test semeiotico per l'afasia e per le funzioni connesse. *Archivio di Psicologia, Neurologia e Psichiatria*, 1960, *21*, 17.

De Renzi, E., & Faglioni, P. L'esame dei disturbi afasici di comprensione orale mediante una versione abbreviata del test dei gettoni. *Rivista di Patologia Nervosa e Mentale*, 1975, *96*, 252-269.

De Renzi, E. & Faglioni, P. Normative data and screening power of a shortened version of the Token Test. *Cortex*, 1978, *14*, 41-49.

De Renzi, E., Faglioni, P., & Previdi, P. Increased susceptibility of aphasics to a distractor task in the recall of verbal commands. *Brain and Language*, 1978, *6*, 14-21.

De Renzi, E., & Vignolo, L. A. The Token Test: A sensitive test to detect receptive disturbances in aphasics. *Brain*, 1962, *85*, 665-678.

Derouesné, J., & Lecours, A. R. Two tests for the study of semantic deficits in aphasia. *International Journal of Mental Health*, 1972, *1*(3), 14-24.

Deutsch, M. The role of social class in language development and cognition. *American Journal of Orthopsychiatry*, 1965, *35*, 78-88.

Dunn, L. M. *Expanded Manual for the Peabody Picture Vocabulary Test.* Circle Pines: American Guidance Service, 1965.

Fitzhugh, K. B., Fitzhugh, L. C., & Reitan, R. M. Wechsler-Bellevue comparisons in groups with "chronic" and "current" lateralized and diffuse brain lesions. *Journal of Consulting Psychology*, 1962, *26*, 306-310.

Gardner, H. The contribution of operativity to naming capacity in aphasic patients. *Neuropsychologia*, 1973, *11*, 213-220

Geschwind, N. Disconnexion syndromes in animals and man (Part I). *Brain*, 1965, *88*, 237-294.

Gleason, J. B., Goodglass, H., Green, E., Ackerman, N., & Hyde, M. R. The retrieval of syntax in Broca's aphasia. *Brain and Language*, 1975, *2*, 451-471.

Goldstein, K. *Language and language disturbances.* New York: Grune & Stratton, 1948.

Goodglass, H., & Baker, E. Semantic field, naming and auditory comprehension in aphasia. *Brain and Language*, 1976, *3*, 359-374.

# REFERENCES

Goodglass, H., & Blumstein, S. (Eds.). *Psycholinguistics and Aphasia.* Baltimore: Johns Hopkins Press, 1973.

Goodglass, H., Blumstein, S., Gleason, J. B., Green, E., Hyde, M., & Statlender, S. *The effect of syntactic encoding on sentence comprehension in aphasia.* Paper presented at the 15th Annual Meeting of the Academy of Aphasia, Montreal, October, 1977.

Goodglass, H., Gleason, J. B., & Hyde, M. Some dimensions of auditory language comprehension in aphasics. *Journal of Speech and Hearing Research,* 1970, *13,* 595-606.

Goodglass, H., & Hunt, J. Grammatical complexity and aphasic speech. *Word,* 1958, *14,* 197-207.

Goodglass, H., & Kaplan, E. *The assessment of aphasia and related disorders.* Philadelphia: Lea & Febiger, 1972.

Gottschaldt, K. Ueber den Einfluss der Erfahrung auf die Wahrnehmung von Figuren. *Psychologische Forschung,* 1929, *12,* 1-87.

Grashey, H. Ueber Aphasie und ihre Beziehungen zur Wahrnehmung. *Archiv für Psychiatrie,* 1885, *16,* 654-688.

Hartje, W., Kerschensteiner, M., Poeck, K., & Orgass, B. A cross-validation study on the Token Test. *Neuropsychologia,* 1973, *11,* 119-121.

Head, H. *Aphasia and kindred disorders of speech.* Cambridge: Cambridge University Press, 1926.

Heilman, K. M., & Scholes, R. J. The nature of comprehension errors in Broca's conduction and Wernicke's aphasics. *Cortex,* 1976, *12,* 258-265.

Holland, A. L., & Sonderman, J. C. Effects of a program based on the Token Test for teaching comprehension skills to aphasics. *Journal of Speech and Hearing Research,* 1974, *17,* 589-598.

Hounsfield, G. N. Computerized transverse axial scanning (tomography). Part 1. Description of system. *British Journal of Radiology,* 1973, *46,* 1016-1022.

Howes, D., & Boller, F. Simple Reaction Time: Evidence for focal impairment from lesions of the right hemisphere. *Brain,* 1975, *98,* 317-332.

Kimura, D. The asymmetry of the human brain. *Scientific American,* 1973, *228,* 70-78.

Kimura, D. Acquisition of a motor skill after left hemisphere damage. *Brain,* 1977, *100,* 527-542.

Kimura, D., & Archibald, Y. Motor functions of the left hemisphere. *Brain,* 1974, *97,* 337-350.

Kirk, S. A., McCarthy, J. J., & Kirk, W. D. *Illinois Test of Psycholinguistic Abilities* (rev. ed.). Urbana: University of Illinois Press, 1968.

Kleist, K. Kriegsverletzungen des Gehirns in ibrer Bedeutung für die Hirnlokalisation und Hirnpathologie. In O. von Schjerning (Ed.), *Handbuch der ärztlichen Erfahrungen im Weltkriege 1914/1918,* Leipzig, *4,* 343, 1922-1934.

Kreindler, A., Gheorghita, N., & Voinescu, I. Analysis of verbal reception of a complex order with three elements in aphasics. *Brain,* 1971, *94,* 375-386.

Kuçera, H., & Francis, W. N. *Computational Analysis of Present-day American English.* Providence: Brown University Press, 1967.

La Pointe, L. L., Horner, J., Liberman, R. J., & Riški, J. E. Assessing patterns of auditory perception and comprehension impairment in aphasia. Paper presented at the 12th Annual Meeting of the Academy of Aphasia, Warrenton, VA. October, 1974.

Leischner, A. Die neuropsychologisch-hirnpathologische Untersuchung. *Archiv für Psychiatrie und Nervenkrankeiten,* 1974, *219,* 53-77.

Lesser, R. Verbal comprehension in aphasia: An English version of three Italian tests. *Cortex,* 1974, *10,* 247-263.

Lesser, R. Verbal and non-verbal memory components in the Token Test. *Neuropsychologia,* 1976, *14,* 79-85.

Lesser, R. *Linguistic Investigations of Aphasia.* London: E. Arnold, 1978.
Lieberman, G. J., & Miller, R. G., Jr. Simultaneous tolerance intervals in regression. *Biometrika*, 1963, *50*, 155-168.
Liepmann, H. *Drei Aufsatze aus dem Apraxiegebiet.* Berlin: S. Karger, 1908.
Liles, B. Z., & Brookshire, R. H. The effects of pause time on auditory comprehension of aphasic subjects. *Journal of Communication Disorders*, 1975, *8*, 221-236.
Locke, J. L., & Deck, J. W. Retrieval failure, rehearsal deficiency and short-term memory loss in the aphasic adult. *Brain and Language*, 1978, *5*, 227-235.
Luria, A. R. *Traumatic aphasia.* The Hague: Mouton, 1970.
Luria, A. R., & Yoduvich, F. I. *Speech and the Development of Mental Processes in the Child.* London: Staples Press, 1959.
Marie, P. La troisième circonvolution frontale ne joue aucun rôle spécial dans la function du langage. *Semaine Médicale*, 1906, *26*, 241-247.
Mazzocchi, F., & Vignolo, L. A. Computer assisted tomography in neuropsychological research: A simple procedure for lesion mapping. *Cortex*, 1978, *14*, 136-166.
McNeil, M. R., & Prescott, T. E. *Revised Token Test.* Baltimore: University Park Press, 1978.
Miller, G. A. *Language and Communication.* New York: McGraw-Hill, 1951.
Noll, J. D., & Randolph, S. R. Auditory semantic, syntactic, and retention errors made by aphasic subjects on the Token Test. *Journal of Communication Disorders*, 1978, *11*, 543-553.
Ombredane, A. *L'aphasie et l'élaboration de la pensée explicite.* Paris: Presse Universitaire de France, 1951.
Orgass, B. *Eine Revision des Token Tests.* Unpublished manuscript, Aachen, 1975.
Orgass, B., & Poeck, K. Clinical validation of a new test for aphasia: An experimental study of the Token Test. *Cortex*, 1966, *2*, 222-243.
Orgass, B., & Poeck, K. Assessment of aphasia by psychometric methods. *Cortex*, 1969, *5*, 317-330.
Parisi, D., & Pizzamiglio, L. Syntactic comprehension in aphasia. *Cortex*, 1970, *6*, 204-215.
Pearson, G. H., Alpers, B. J., & Weisenburg, T. Aphasia: A study of normal control cases. *Archives of Neurology and Psychiatry*, 1928, *19*, 281-295.
Peck, D. J. *The effects of presentation rates on the auditory comprehension of learning disabled children.* Unpublished master's thesis, University of Florida, 1977.
Pizzamiglio, L., & Appicciafuoco, A. Semantic comprehension in aphasia. *Journal of Communication Disorders*, 1971, *3*, 280-288.
Poeck, K., Kerschensteiner, M., & Hartje, W. A quantitative study on language understanding in fluent and nonfluent aphasia. *Cortex*, 1972, *8*, 299-304.
Poeck, K., Hartje, W., Kerschensteiner, M., & Orgass, B. Sprachvertandnisstorungen bei aphasischen und nichtaphasischen Hirnkranken. *Deutsche Medizinische Wochenschrift*, 1973, *98*, 139-147.
Poeck, K., Kerschensteiner, M., Stachowiak, F. J., & Huber, W. Die amnestische Aphasie; klinisches Bild und uberlegungen zur neurolinguistischen Struktur. *Journal of Neurology*, 1974, *207*, 1-17.
Poeck, K., Orgass, B., Kerschensteiner, M., & Hartje, W. A qualitative study of Token Test performance in aphasic and non-aphasic brain-damaged patients. *Neuropsychologia*, 1974, *12*, 49-54.
Proust, A. De l'aphasie. *Archives générales de Médecine*, 1872, *28*, 147-166; 303-318; 653-685.
Quadfasel, F. Ein Beitrag zum motorischen Verhalten Aphasischer. *Monatschrift fur Psychiatrie und Neurologie*, 1931, *80*, 151-188.
Rieger, C. Beschreibung der Intelligenzstorungen in Folge einer Hirnverletzung und Entwurf zu einer allgemein andwendbaren Methode der Intelligenz Profung. *Ver-*

handlungen der Physikalischen-medizinischen Gesellschaft zur Wurzburg, 1888-1890, 22, 65-134; 23, 95-150.

Saffran, E. M., & Marin, O. S. M. Immediate memory for word lists and sentences in a patient with deficient auditory short-term memory. *Brain and Language*, 1975, 2, 420-433.

Salvatore, A. P. An investigation of the effects of pause duration on sentence comprehension by aphasic subjects. Paper presented at the Annual Meeting of the American Speech and Hearing Association, Washington, D.C., 1975.

Salvatore, A. P., Strait, M., & Brookshire, R. Effects of patient characteristics on delivery of the Token Test commands by experienced and inexperienced examiners. *Journal of Communication Disorders*, 1978, 11, 65-78.

Schuell, H. Some dimensions of aphasic impairment in adults considered in relationship to investigations of language disturbances in children. *British Journal of Disorders of Communication*, 1966, 1, 33-47.

Schwartz, M. F., Saffran, E. M., & Marin, O. S. M. The nature of the comprehension deficit in agrammatic aphasia. Paper presented at the annual meeting of the International Neuropsychological Society, Minneapolis, February, 1978.

Scolaro, C., & Flowers, C. *Variables which affect aphasic persons' ability to follow oral commands.* Paper presented at Annual Meeting of the American Speech and Hearing Association, Chicago, 1977.

Scotti, G., & Spinnler, H. Colour imperception in unilateral hemisphere-damaged patients. *Journal of Neurology, Neurosurgery and Psychiatry*, 1970. 33. 22-28.

Shallice, T., & Butterworth, B. Short-term memory impairment and spontaneous speech. *Neuropsychologia*, 1977, 15, 729-735.

Shewan, C. M., & Canter, G. J. Effects of vocabulary, syntax and sentence length in auditory comprehension in aphasic patients. *Cortex*, 1971, 7, 209-226.

Siegal, S. *Nonparametric Statistics for the Behavioral Sciences.* New York: McGraw-Hill, 1956.

Sipos, J., & Tägert, J. Kurzverfahren zur Erfassung von aphasischen Störungen. *Der Nervenarzt*, 1972, 43, 207-211.

Spellacy, F. J., & Spreen, O. A short form of the Token Test. *Cortex*, 1969, 5, 390-397.

Sperry, R. W. Lateral specialization in the surgically separated hemispheres. In F. O. Schmidt & F. G. Worden (Eds.), The Neurosciences: Third study program. Cambridge, Massachusetts: MIT Press. Pp. 5-19.

Spreen, O., & Benton, A. L. *Neurosensory Center Comprehensive Examination for Aphasia.* British Columbia: University of Victoria, 1969.

Stockwell, R. P., Schachter, P., & Partee, B. H. *The major syntactic structures of English.* New York: Holt, Rinehart, & Winston. 1973.

Swisher, L. P., & Sarno, M. T. Token Test scores of three matched patient groups—left-brain damaged with aphasia, right-brain-damaged without aphasia and non-brain-damaged. *Cortex*, 1969, 5, 264-273.

Tägert, J., Chock, D., Niklas, J., Sandvoss, G., & Sipos, J. Linguistische Funktionstörungen bei Patienten mit rechthirnigen Läsionen. *Der Nervenartz*, 1975, 46, 249-255.

Tallal, P. Perceptual and linguistic factors in the language impairment of developmental dysphasics: An experimental investigation with the Token Test. *Cortex*, 1975, 11, 196-205.

Thorndike, E. L., & Lorge, I. *The Teacher's Word Book of 30,000 Words.* New York: Teachers College Press, 1944.

Toppin, C. J., & Brookshire, R. H. Effects of response delay and Token relocation on Token Test performance of aphasic subjects. *Journal of Communication Disorders*, 1978, 11, 65-78.

Van Dongen, H. R., & van Harskamp, F. The Token Test: A preliminary evaluation of a method to detect aphasia. *Psychiatria, Neurologia Neurochirurgia,* 1972, *75,* 129-134.

Vilkki, J., & Laitinen, L. V. Differential effects of left and right ventrolateral thalamotomy on receptive and expressive verbal performances and face matching. *Neuropsychologia,* 1974, *12,* 11-19.

Warrington, E. K., Logue, V., & Pratt, R. T. C. The anatomical localization of selective impairment of auditory verbal short-term memory. *Neuropsychologia,* 1971, *9,* 377-387.

Weisenburg, T., & McBride, K. E. *Aphasia: A clinical and psychological study.* New York: Commonwealth Fund, 1935.

Wepman, J. M., Bock, R. D., Jones, L. V., & Van Pelt, D. Psycholinguistic study of aphasia: A revision of the concept of anomia. *Journal of Speech and Hearing Disorders,* 1956, *21,* 468-477.

Wernicke, C. *Der aphasische Symptomenkomplex.* Breslau: Cohn & Weigert, 1874.

West, J. A. Auditory comprehension in aphasic adults. *Archives of Physical Medicine and Rehabilitation,* 1973, *54,* 78-86.

Whitaker, H. A. *On the representation of language in the human brain.* Edmonton: Linguistic Research, 1971.

Whitaker, H. A., & Noll, J. D. Some linguistic parameters of the Token Test. *Neuropsychologia,* 1972, *10,* 395-404.

Whitaker, H. A., & Selnes, O. A. Token Test Measures of Language Comprehension in Normal Children and Aphasic Patients. In A. Caramazza & E. B. Zurif (Eds.), *Language Acquisition and Language Breakdown.* Baltimore: Johns Hopkins Press, 1978.

Whitaker, H., & Whitaker, H. A. Linguistic Theory and Speech Pathology. *Journal of Minnesota Speech & Hearing Association,* 1972, *11,* 51-56.

Whitney, J. L. Developing aphasics' use of compensatory strategies. Paper presented at the Annual Meeting of the American Speech and Hearing Association, Washington, D.C., 1975.

Winer, B. J. *Statistical Principles in Experimental Design.* New York: McGraw-Hill, 1972.

Yorkston, K. M., Marshall, R. C., & Butler, M. Imposed delay of response: Effects on aphasics' auditory comprehension of visually and nonvisually cued material. *Perceptual & Motor Skills,* 1977, *44,* 647-655.

Zaidel, E. Linguistic competence and related functions in the right cerebral hemisphere of man following commissurotomy and hemispherectomy (Doctoral Dissertation, California Institute of Technology). *Dissertation Abstracts International,* 1973, *34,* 2350B. (University Microfilms No. 73-26, 481.)

Zaidel, E. A technique for presenting lateralized visual input with prolonged exposure. *Vision Research,* 1975, *15,* 283-289. (a)

Zaidel, E. The case of the elusive right hemisphere. Paper presented at the 13th annual meeting of the Academy of Aphasia, Victoria, B.C., Oct. 7, 1975. (b)

Zaidel, E. Language, dichotic listening and the disconnected hemispheres. In D. O. Walter, L. Rogers, & J. M. Finzi-Fried (Eds.), *Conference on Human Brain Function.* Brain Information Service/BRI Publications Office, UCLA, 103-110, 1976. (a)

Zaidel, E. Auditory vocabulary of the right hemisphere following brain bisection or hemidecortication. *Cortex,* 1976, *12,* 191-211. (b)

Zaidel, E. Unilateral auditory language comprehension on the Token Test following cerebral commissurotomy and hemispherectomy. *Neuropsychologia,* 1977, *15,* 1-18.

Zaidel, E. Auditory language comprehension in the right hemisphere following cerebral commissurotomy and hemispherectomy: A comparison with child language and aphasia. In A. Caramazza & E. B. Zurif (Eds.), *Language Acquisition and Language Breakdown: Parallels and Divergencies.* Baltimore: Johns Hopkins University Press, 1978. Pp. 229-275. (a)

Zaidel, E. Lexical organization in the right hemisphere. In P. Buser & A. Rougeul-Buser (Eds.), *Cerebral Correlates of Conscious Experience*. Amsterdam: Elsevier, 1978. Pp. 177–197. (b)

Zaidel, E. Concepts of cerebral dominance in the split brain. In P. Buser & A. Rougeul-Buser (Eds.), *Cerebral Correlates of Conscious Experience*. Amsterdam: Elsevier, 1978. Pp. 263–284. (c)

Zaidel, E. The split and half brains as models of congenital language disability. In C. L. Ludlow & M. E. Doran-Quine (Eds.), NINCDS Symposium on *The Neurological Bases of Language Disorders in Children: Methods and Directions for Research* (NINCDS Monograph). Washington, D.C.: Government Printing Office, in press, 1978. (d)

Zaidel, E. Performance on the ITPA following cerebral commissurotomy and hemispherectomy. *Neuropsychologia*, in press.

Zaidel, E., Zaidel, D., & Sperry, R. W. Left and right intelligence: Unilateral performance on the book and board forms of Raven's Progressive Matrices following brain bisection and hemidortication. Submitted for publication, 1978.

Zurif, E. B., Caramazza, A., & Myerson, R. Grammatical judgments of agrammatic aphasics. *Neuropsychologia*, 1972, *10*, 405–417.

# Subject Index

Auditory comprehension
  anatomical substrate for, 161, 163–167
  historical tests of, 3–11
  lexical, semantic, and syntactic aspects of, 45–46, 63, 89–106
  supramodal deficit and, 112–113

Head aphasia tests, 7–9, 15

Marie Paper Test, 6–7, 16

Ombredane aphasia tests, 9–11

Performance on Token Test
  aphasics and, 24–26, 38–40, 52–54, 57–58, 61–62, 79, 109–110, 163–167
  CT-scan verified lesions, 163–167
  fluent and nonfluent compared, 52–54, 57–58, 61–62
  left hemisphere damage, 38–40, 52–54

  unspecified brain damage, 24–26, 79, 109–110
  children and, 41–42, 127–129
  economically disadvantaged, 127–129
  commissurotomized and hemispherectomized patients, 140–153
  laterality effects, 140–146
  long-term changes, 146–151
  short-term variability, 151–153
  nonaphasics, 40
  left hemisphere damage, 40
  right hemisphere damage, 40

Token Test
  aphasics and, see Performance on Token Test
  children and, see Performance on Token Test
  commissurotomized and hemispherectomized patients and, see Performance on Token Test

Token Test (*continued*)
  discriminative power, 43, 52–53, 60–61, 63–64, 111–113, 135, 177–179
  error analyses, 26–28, 55–61, 79–82, 82–84, 176–177
  item lists, 44, 67–69, 131–132, 158–159
  linguistic analyses of, 89–106, 172–175
    case grammars, 95–105
    syntax, 93–95
    word frequency, 90–93
  memory factors and, 64–65, 74–75, 80–82, 93–94, 173–175
  nonaphasics and, *see* Performance on Token Test
  original description of, 20–24
  other tests and, 54–55, 110–111, 174
  performance on, *see* Performance on Token Test
  recovery from aphasia and, 153–154
  revised forms, 34–37, 50–51, 63–64, 75–78, 79–80, 108–109, 137–140
    compared with standard, 34–35, 63–64, 79–80, 109
    contact lens administration, 137–140
    lexical and syntactic, 50–51
    real objects, 75–78
    short, 35–37
    written, 108–109
  scoring, 39, 52, 126, 140, 155–159
  training programs based on, 122–124
  verified brain damage and, 163–167, 179–180

Weisenburg and McBride aphasia tests, 9, 17

**NO LONGER THE PROPERTY
OF THE
UNIVERSITY OF RI LIBRARY**